Recent Results
in Cancer Research

149

Managing Editors
P. M. Schlag, Berlin · H.-J. Senn, St. Gallen

Associate Editors
V. Diehl, Cologne · D.M. Parkin, Lyon
M.F. Rajewsky, Essen · R. Rubens, London
M. Wannenmacher, Heidelberg

Founding Editor
P. Rentchnik, Geneva

Springer

Berlin
Heidelberg
New York
Barcelona
Hong Kong
London
Milan
Paris
Singapore
Tokyo

B. Thürlimann

Bisphosphonates in Clinical Oncology

The Development of Pamidronate

With 24 Figures and 15 Tables

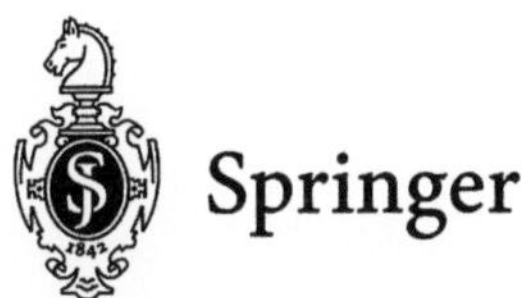

Springer

Dr. med. Beat Thürlimann
Kantonsspital St. Gallen
Klinik C für Innere Medizin
Abteilung für Onkologie und Hämatologie
CH-9007 St. Gallen

ISBN-13:978-3-642-64148-0   e-ISBN-13:978-3-642-59845-6
DOI: 10.1007/978-3-642-59845-6

ISSN 0080-0015

Library of Congress Cataloging-in-Publication Data
Bisphosphonates in clinical oncology: the development in pamidronate/B. Thürlimann
(ed.). p. cm. – (Recent results in cancer research, ISSN 0080-0015; 149). Includes biblio-
graphical references and index.ISBN-13:978-3-642-64148-0(hardcover: alk.paper).1.Disodium
pamidronate. 2. Bones–Cancer–Chemotherapy. 3. Diphosphonates–Therapeutic use. I.
Thürlimann, B. (Beat), 1955–. II. Series. [DNLM: 1. Diphosphonates-pharmacology.
2. Antineoplastic Agents–pharmacology. 3. Hypercalcemia–drug therapy. 4. Bone Neoplasms–drug therapy. 5. Bone Neoplasms–secondary. 6. Bone and Bones–physiology. [W1 RE106P v. 149 1998/QZ 267 B6157 1998] RC261R35 vol. 149 [RC280.B6]
616.99′4 s [616.99′4061]–DC21 DNLM/DLC for Library of Congress.

The use of general descriptive names, registered names, trademarks, etc. in this publication
does not imply, even in the absence of a specific statement, that such names are exempt
from the relevant protective laws and regulations and therefore free for general use.

Product liability: The publisher cannot guarantee the accuracy of any information about
dosage and application contained in this book. In every individual case the user must
check such information by consulting the relevant literature.

Production: PRO EDIT GmbH, D-69126 Heidelberg
Typesetting: K+V Fotosatz GmbH, D-64743 Beerfelden

SPIN 10643981   19/3133-5 4 3 2 1 0 – Printed on acid-free paper

To Anne, who made all this possible.
To Annatina, Christian, and Andres,
who had enough patience with their father.

Preface

The book gives an overview of the clinical developments in the use of bisphosphonates in clinical oncology. The first part presents the composition, physiology, and pathophysiology of bone. Next is a section giving insight into mechanisms of bone resorption, bone formation, and bone remodeling, a field in which I was most influenced by O.L.M. Bijvoet and H. Fleisch. The second part summarizes the pharmacological treatments for disorders of bone remodeling. The clinical aspects of tumor-induced hypercalcemia and its management are described in detail, including our first prospective randomized crossover study testing pamidronate versus mithramycin. The bisphosphonates were introduced in clinical oncology by endocrinologists. The same was true for our institution in 1986, when P. Burckhardt proposed testing pamidronate in the above-mentioned trial in his institution (CHUV) and in our department. The impressive results obtained in the hypercalcemia trial stimulated our interest, and we actively investigated the use of pamidronate to counteract osteolytic bone destruction in cancer patients. These investigations are presented and discussed in the third part. They represent the interdisciplinary work involving many co-workers of the Department of Internal Medicine C and other institutes of the Interdisciplinary Oncology Center St. Gallen (IOSG), which I was privileged to chair for 10 years. Initially, a pharmacokinetic study was performed in order to optimize and facilitate the administration of the drug to patients with malignant osteolytic bone disease. The results of this study established the basis for and the safety of repeated pamidronate infusions and led to the dose-escalation and finally to the randomized dose-finding studies. At the same time, we participated in the clinical development of pamidronate within the large multicenter phase-III study in patients with breast cancer receiving their first chemotherapy for advanced disease. In collaboration with the *Institut für Management im Gesundheitswesen* of the University of St. Gallen and based on the clinical results of this study, we developed a model for evaluation of the cost-benefit of pamidronate treatment in the group of Swiss patients. A summary of cost-benefit considerations of our last double-blind dose-effect study is also added. Finally, recent developments are reported, including a short description of our participation in the clinical development of ibandronate and early experiences with adjuvant therapy.

The first part of this booklet provides an overview of the mechanisms of physiological bone remodeling, their disorders, and possibilities of therapeutic interventions. The results of our studies presented in the second part may contribute to the knowledge of pamidronate and of how to best use the drug.

November 1998   *Dr. med. Beat Thürlimann*

Acknowledgements

The development of bisphosphonates for use in oncology is a good example of interdisciplinary teamwork. The advances made at our cancer center have been possible only with the cooperation of many health-care professionals working together to achieve a common goal.

I am indebted to Professor Dr. Hans-Jörg Senn, formerly Head of the Department of Internal Medicine C, and now Scientific Director of the Center for Early Cancer Detection and Prevention in St. Gallen, Switzerland for creating an environment which made clinical research an affair of daily routine, by recommending and administering experimental drugs as the best available treatment to cancer patients. He initiated research into bisphosphonates at the very beginning of their development in the field of clinical oncology and encouraged me continuously to conduct all these studies and to communicate their results.

The clinical research fellows who worked in our department from 1985 on and helped to implement and conduct the studies within the daily routine are Drs. Alexander Radziwil, Fabia Weisser, Liza Bacchus, and Dieter Köberle. I am also grateful to the other members of our team from the Interdisciplinary Oncology Center St. Gallen (IOSG): Dr. Rudolf Morant, Head of the Division of Oncology/Hematology, who supported the clinical conduct of the trial and helped with the analysis of data; Dr. Renato Waldburger, who conducted the first clinical study testing pamidronate versus mithramycin in tumor-induced hypercalcemia 10 years ago; Dr. Hanna Engler and Prof. Walter Riesen, from the Institute of Hematology and Chemistry (IKCH), who made the laboratory investigations of new bone turnover markers possible; the research nurses Jacqueline Meier and Christel Böhme, who performed the blinding of the last study and administered many bisphosphonate infusions.

I also want thank the people of Novartis, formerly Ciba Geigy Headquarters, and Ciba Geigy Pharma Switzerland, Basel, Switzerland, who supported our research of pamidronate throughout the 10-year period: Professor Hobitz and Dr. Ch. Nadjafi, who initiated the research, and Dr. J. Gloor for his continuous support; Dr. V.V. Maly from the Statistical Office of Ciba Headquarters, who analyzed our first pamidronate study; Dr. R. van der Giessen and Werner Osterwalder from the Central Product Management of the Pharma Division of Ciba Geigy Headquarters, who always had an open ear for our needs.

We also thank Dr. de Jong from the Pharmaco-Economic Department of Ciba-Geigy Headquarters and Dr. B. Horisberger and Dr. U. Gessner from the Research Group on Management in the Health System of the University of St. Gallen, Switzerland for their input in the pharmacoeconomic aspects of the trials.

In addition, I am grateful for the statistical advice given by Dr. Ruedi Maibach, Chief Statistician of the Coordination Center of the Swiss Group for Clinical Cancer Research (SAKK, Berne, Switzerland). Marisa Bacchi, also from the Statistical Office of the SAKK Coordination Center, helped us in analyzing the data from our first randomized pamidronate study in malignant osteolytic bone disease.

I thank Dr. Martin and Pamela Chasen, Santon Oncology Center, Johannesburg, South Africa, for the critical review and the linguistic improvement of the manuscript.

Finally, our thanks are also due to Mrs. J. Blank and Mrs. C. Würsdörfer from the Department of Internal Medicine C, Kantonsspital, St. Gallen, Switzerland for their secretarial help.

Contents

Physiology and Pathophysiology of Bone

Introduction

Remodeling and turnover of bone is a key phenomenon in bone physiology. The mechanisms which control the remodeling process and its regulation will clarify not only such local phenomenona as malignant osteolytic bone disease and healing of fractures but also the pathophysiology of age-related bone loss and other systemic bone disorders. Abnormalities in bone remodeling occur in common diseases. Age-related bone loss and osteoporosis are associated with considerable morbidity and are a major public health issue in Western societies. Both affect more than 25% of aging women and about 5–10% of the male population. Other systemic bone diseases with increased bone resorption are also more common than previously believed. Paget's disease affects up to 3% of the population over the age of 40 in Western countries. Primary hyperparathyroidism has also been recognized as a common disease, now that serum calcium has been included in the routine screening of blood chemistry examination in many countries; the prevalence is estimated at 1/1000 adults in the United States. Malignant osteolytic bone disease is also a common disorder. Breast cancer in women and prostate cancer in men are among the malignant diseases with the highest incidence in Western countries; e.g., in the 1990s, about 325,000 women have died every year of breast cancer worldwide, accounting for 16% of all cancer deaths among women in developed countries and 11% in developing countries. The disease affects more women in most industrialized countries than in other countries, and it is the third most frequent cancer among the population as whole. One in every ten women in Switzerland is expected to develop breast cancer during her lifetime, and half of them will die from it (Coleman et al. 1993; Levy et al. 1996).

Although these disorders are common we do not fully understand either the mechanisms that are responsible for the control of normal bone remodeling, its coordination and maintenance of balance or those responsible for the imbalance of bone remodeling which characterises the above-mentioned diseases. However, some therapeutic progress has been made, and the recent development of useful bisphosphonate provides an important tool for the clinician to positively influence the pathophysiology and the complications associated with imbalanced bone remodeling.

Natural History of the Skeleton

Bone mass reaches its maximum about 10 years after linear growth stops and probably begins to decrease in the 4th decade, declining to half its maximum by the time a person reaches the age of 80. The highest values of bone mineral density are measured in the 3rd and 4th decades; higher values are measured in men than in women and lower values in Caucasians than in the African population. However, women of all ethnic groups show an additional accelerated phase of bone loss about 10 years after menopause. The menopause-associated bone loss accounts for about half of the total bone loss associated with aging. It is estimated that 35% of cortical bone and 50% of trabecular bone is lost in women. The male population is calculated to lose about two thirds of the amount lost by women (Mazess 1982; Riggs et al. 1986).

Cortical bone and trabecular bone do not change with age in exactly the same way, and so they should probably be considered as two separate compartments. This might be due to the fact that trabecular bone has a greater surface and its modulation is influenced to a higher degree by the paracrine effect of osteotropic cytokines, which are released by cells of the marrow cavity. On the other hand, cortical bone remodeling might be more influenced by systemic osteotropic hormones in an endocrine fashion such as parathyroid hormone and 1,25-dihydroxyvitamin D_3. It is still not clear whether there is a similar accelerated phase of bone loss in both trabecular and cortical bone after the menopause. Different measuring techniques of bone mineral density have given different answers. The overall fracture threshold is estimated to be reached between the ages of 60 and 75 years in women and after 85 years of age in men. The proportion of cortical and trabecular bone in various parts of the skeleton and mechanical properties such as stiffness and strength of the bone will determine the predilection of localization for fractures with a given mechanical impact on a part of the body (Smith et al. 1975).

Trabecular bone is prominent in the vertebral column and amounts to more than 66% of the total bone in the lumber spine, which is also the most common site of fractures associated with osteoporosis. The abnormality in the bone-remodeling process, and particularly the loss of trabecular bone associated with menopause, may at least partly explain the predisposition to this type of fracture. The intertrochanteric area of the femur is composed of about 50% cortical and 50% trabecular bone; the neck of the femur is about 75% cortical and 25% trabecular bone. The higher mechanical impact in this part of the body might explain also the large number of fractures that occur in this part of the skeleton. A similar content of cortical and trabecular bone is seen at the distal end of the radius, whereas in the mid radius more than 95% of the bone is cortical. The diameter and the composition of trabecular and cortical bone of the radius might also explain the greater incidence of distal radius fractures compared with the relatively rare events in the mid radius.

Cortical Bone

Cortical bone constitutes about 85% of the total human skeleton. The volume of cortical bone is regulated by endosteal resorption, by the formation of periosteal bone, and by remodeling within the haversian canals. Periosteal bone formation continues throughout life and increases the mechanical properties of bone, not only by simply counteracting bone resorption but also by increasing the diameter of cortical bone. Cortical bone loss begins around the age of 40 and is accelerated 5–10 years after menopause. This accelerated phase of cortical bone loss continues for 15 years and then gradually slows down. Estrogen replacement therapy can prevent menopause-associated bone loss. Bone loss is increased in women with artificial menopause, e.g., in younger women with breast cancer and chemotherapy-induced amenorrhea (Saarto et al. 1995).

Cortical bone loss is the major predisposing factor for hip fractures. As mentioned above, cortical bone remodeling is controlled mainly by endocrine factors. It is thus not surprising that cortical bone is the main target of bone resorption in patients with primary hyperparathyroidism.

Trabecular Bone

Despite the fact that trabecular bone constitutes only 15% of the skeleton, the abnormalities in remodeling that occur will determine the incidence of osteoporosis and frequency of fractures associated with it. It remains unclear whether tabecular bone loss starts earlier (Riggs et al. 1986; Genant et al. 1982). However, is has been suggested that menopause-associated trabecular bone loss is less prominent than the accelerated cortical bone loss at the time of menopause (Riggs and Melton 1986). The loss of trabecular bone with aging and the loss of its mechanical strength is not caused mainly by generalized resorption of the bone plates; it is due rather to a complete perforation and fragmentation of trabeculae (Parfitt et al. 1983; Kleerekoper et al. 1985). The mean thickness of trabecular bone plates is approximately 100–150 µm, whereas osteoclasts cause resorption defects of about 50–100 µm during the normal remodeling process. An increased number of remodeling units or activation of an existing remodeling site – for example, caused by estrogen deficiency after the menopause – can lead to focal perforation of trabecular bone plates. This perforation may lead to the lack of a basis of support for new bone formation even when osteoblasts are stimulated to form new bone. This also means that a bone plate which once has broken cannot be restored and cannot contribute to restoration of the impaired mechanical properties of the bone. The perforation of bone plates, once it has started, places the remaining still normal or already weakened bone in a disadvantageous structural position and increases the risk of fractures of those bone plates. This vicious circle leads to an advanced stage of weakening of the mechanical properties of mainly trabecular bone at a point in time when the consequences of this process only begin to become clinically apparent or can be seen on plain X-rays. It is therefore also easy to understand that the breakdown of conductivity of horizontal bone plates cannot be repaired by currently applied osteoporosis therapy. This may also explain the limited clinical success of present-day osteoporosis treatment and why it is more advantageous to take a preventive approach, rather than attempting to restore adequate mechanical properties to trabecular bone. Osteolytic bone disease due to malignancy takes place also in the trabecular compartment. It originates from malignant cells which lodge in the marrow cavity and produce local factors that stimulate osteoclasts on the trabecular endosteal surfaces of cortical bone. Evidence of bone resorbing activity and the formation of osteoclast-stimulating factors was found more than 20 years ago (Mundy et al. 1974a,b).

Composition of Bone

Essentially, the composition of bone is 65% mineral (hydroxyapatite), 35% matrix cells (osteoblasts, osteocytes, osteoclasts), and water. Bone mineral is basically hydroxyapatite, but it has many other chemical constituents. These are either incorporated in the crystals or adsorbed on the surface. Some compounds such as tetracyclines and bisphosphonates have a special affinity for crystalline surfaces. Tetracyclines are used to label newly formed bone.

In fact, the amount of newly formed bone can be estimated by measuring the distance between two lines of tetracycline deposition seen in bone biopsies when tetracycline has been administered to an individual twice at aknown time interval. The bone-seeking properties of bisphosphonates have already been used in nuclear medicine to visualize hot spots of bone formation by scintigraphy.

About 90% of the bone matrix is collagen, which is arranged in a complex three-dimensional structure. This structure is important mainly for the tensile strength of the bone. The urinary excretion and plasma levels of degradation products are used to estimate bone resorption.

Bone Cells

Osteoblasts. Osteoblasts are derived from mesenchymal stem cells which are located in the bone marrow. They synthesize bone matrix directionally at the surface of bone. This matrix is later calcified extracellularly. The layer of demineralized bone matrix under the osteoblasts decreases when bone formation is diminished but increases when bone mineralization is delayed. In osteomalacia, where there is almost complete loss of mineralization, wide layers of demineralized bone matrix can be seen and are the hallmark of the diagnosis.

Osteocytes. When osteoblasts stop matrix synthesis they become embedded within the bone and are called osteocytes. This phenomenon is still little understood. It has been suggested that they are involved in maintaining homeostasis of plasma calcium and in the adaptation of bone in response to mechanical influences.

Osteoclasts. Osteoclasts are derived from hematopoietic cells of the granulocyte-macrophage lineage. Osteoclasts are usually large, multinucleated cells which are frequently situated in Howship's lacunae. They resorb bone by attachment to cell membrane receptors which recognize specific peptide sequences of the matrix. The bone mineral is then dissolved by secretion of H^+ ions, and various proteolytic enzymes destroy the bone matrix. Among these enzymes, cathepsins and collagens are the best known. Bone resorption is modulated by the production of new osteoblasts and the activation of mature osteoclasts. These processes are under the control of osteoblast-lineage cells. A wide range of hormones and cytokines also influence bone resorption.

Factors Regulating Calcium Homeostasis and Bone Resorption/Bone Formation

The plasma calcium concentration is usually kept within a narrow range throughout the animal world and also in man. This constancy is explained by the importance of free extracellular calcium for many biological processes. Total serum calcium is usually kept around 2.3±0.3 mmol/l. About 40% of calcium is bound to serum proteins, 10% to filterable ions. About half of the serum calcium is ionized, and plasma calcium is thus approximately 1.25–1.40 mmol/l. This fraction of ionized calcium (and not total calcium) is closely controlled. Many factors influence calcium homeostasis through complicated mechanisms. How these work together to maintain normal plasma calcium is not fully known. Mundy (1989) proposed a model which is consistent with the available data and is accepted by the majority of endocrinologists, nephrologists, and osteologists: The two major hormones which maintain calcium homeostasis are parathyroid hormone (PTH) and 1,25-dihydroxyvitamin (vitamin D_3). PTH is more important for rapid effects on plasma calcium, whereas vitamin D_3 is more important for its long-term effects. There is a basic level of plasma calcium which is maintained by exchange of calcium between bone fluid, bone surface, and the extracellular fluid that is independent of hormonal activity. Complete absence of PTH or vitamin D_3 does not therefore lead to complete disappearance of calcium from the extracellular fluid. PTH and vitamin D_3 are necessary to raise the basic plasma calcium level of 1.25–1.40 mmol/l to a normal range of approximately 2.3 mmol/l. Oscillations within the normal range are dampened by the above-mentioned hormone-independent bone/extracellular fluid exchange and also by increasing or decreasing levels of PTH and vitamin D_3. These hormones are regulated by negative feedback loops. PTH secretion is not further enhanced or depressed by changes of plasma calcium concentrations outside the range of approximately 1.9–2.9 mmol/l. At these extremes the bone fluid exchange mechanism may be the most important factor for correction of serum calcium concentration. This model is also consistent with the concept of set point and error correction. When a "normal" range for plasma calcium for an individual is concerned, this normal range reflects the set point. It cannot be absolutely measured, but it is estimated in a normal individual from a mean of serial measurements of plasma calcium. This set point is most probably, at least in part, genetically determined, since mean plasma calcium varies little between members of the same family. In conclusion, the set point is the absolute plasma calcium concentration which the homeostatic mechanism attempts to maintain.

Of the hormones that regulate calcemia, the most important is PTH, which acts on three target organs. It increases bone resorption and intestinal absorption of calcium, although indirectly through an elevation of vitamin D_3. It also increases renal tubular reabsorption of calcium. The secretion of PTH is rapidly modulated and inversely correlated to calcemia and therefore provides an excellent, rapidly working negative feedback mechanism. Vitamin D_3 increases intestinal calcium absorption and bone resorption. Its production is stimulated by low plasma calcium. However, PTH is modulated and acts within minutes, whereas vitamin D_3 requires hours to days to exert its influence on calcemia. Calcitonin inhibits bone destruction and can therefore be used in diseases with increased bone resorption. Its relevance in human beings for calcium homeostasis has not yet been established, however. Details of calcium homeostasis are described extensively elsewhere (Mundy 1989).

References

Coleman MP, Esteve J, Daniecki P, Aslan A, Renard H (1993) Trends in cancer: incidence and mortality. IARC ISC Publ 121

Genant HK, Cann CE, Ettinger B, et al (1982) Quantitative computed tomography of vertebral spongiosia: a sensitive method for detecting early bone loss after oophorectomy. Ann Intern Med 97:699–705

Kleerekoper M, Villanueva AR, Stanciu J, et al (1985) The role of 3 dimensional trabecular microstructure in the pathogenesis of vertebral compression fractures. Calcif Tissue Int 37:594–597

Levy F, La Vecchia C, Schüler G, Fopp M, Tschopp A (1996) Occurrence of breast cancer: facts and trends. The National Cancer Control Program: Breast Cancer. Swiss Federal Office of Public Health and Swiss Cancer League, Bern, Switzerland, pp 5–7

Mazess RB (1982) On aging bone loss. Clin Orthop 165:239–252

Mundy GR (1989) Calcium homeostasis: hypercalcemia and hypocalcemia. Martin/Dunitz, London

Mundy GR, Luben RA, Raisz LG, et al (1974a) Bone resorbing activity in supernatants from lymphoid cell lines. N Engl J Med 290:867–871

Mundy GR, Raisz LG, Cooper RA, et al (1974b) Evidence for the secretion of an osteoclast stimulating factor in myeloma. N Engl J Med 291:1041–1046

Parfitt AM, Mathews CHE, Villanueva AR, et al (1983) Relationship between surface, volume and thickness of iliac trabecular bone in aging and in osteoporosis. J Clin Invest 72:1396–1409

Riggs BL, Melton LI III (1986) Involutional osteoporosis. N Engl J Med 314:1676–1686

Riggs BL, Wahner HW, Dunn WL, et al (1981) Differential changes in bone mineral density of the appendicular and axial skeleton with aging: relationship to spinal osteoporosis. J Clin Invest 67:328–335

Riggs BL, Wahner HW, Melton LJ III, et al (1986) Rates of bone loss in the axial and appendicular skeletons of women: evidence of substantial vertebral bone loss prior to menopause. J Clin Invest 77:1487–1491

Saarto T, Blomqvist C, Välimäki M, Mäkelä P, Elmoa L (1995) Clodronate increases bone mineral density in early breast cancer patients: a randomised study. Bone 17:617

Smith DM, Khariri MRA, Johnston CC jr (1975) The loss of bone mineral with aging and its relationship to risk of fracture. J Clin Invest 56:311–318

Bone Resorption

Introduction

The mature bone-resorbing cell is the osteoclast, although other cells such as osteocytes, monocytes, tumor cells, and even osteoblasts may also resorb bone. Osteocytic osteolysis may be due to expansion of the lacunae in which osteocytes are embedded and which have been described by histologists who examined light-microscopic sections. However, scanning electron microscopy indicated that it is unlikely that osteocytes cause osteolysis (Jones et al. 1985). Monocytes and macrophages have been shown to degrade devitalized bone (Kahn et al. 1978; Mundy et al. 1977). These findings support the hypothesis that monocytes and osteoclasts are differentiated cells which arise from a common lineage. Tumor cells also resorb devitalized bone in vitro (Elion and Mundy 1987). On the other hand, no resorption pits were seen when monocytes, macrophages, or tumor cells lay on bone surfaces (Boyde et al. 1986). It has also been suggested that osteoblasts may act as helper cells of osteoclasts by preparing the bone surface. Although cells other than osteoclasts are involved in bone resorption, it is unlikely that they play a major role. The multinucleated osteoclast is the primary bone-resorbing cell. No single criterion is available that is pathognomonic for the osteoclast. Up to this point, it has not been convincingly shown that any kind of method, including immunohistochemical approaches, can specifically identify osteoclasts. However, the presence of 23C6 antibody and calcitonin receptors is helpful, and they are widely used as markers of the osteoclasts (Horton and Davies 1989). A model for osteoclast formation has shown that the osteoclast has a common progenitor with monocytes and macrophages.

Mechanisms of Local Bone Resorption

The osteoclast resorbs bone from the lacunae and then moves across to the bone surfaces to resorb further areas of bone. There is no resorption during periods of locomotion. When the osteoclast eventually stops moving it usually starts to resorb bone. Bone resorption is mediated mainly by proteolytic enzymes and by hydrogen ion secretion into the localized environment under the ruffled border of the osteoclast. These hydrogen ions are produced by the carbonic anhydrase type II and pumped across the ruffled border by a proton pump. New insight has been gained into the molecular mechanism for transport of protons from the cytosol to the ruffled border by the vacuole ATPase. Disruption at any step of this pathway will result in incompetent osteoclasts and may cause osteopetrosis. It has been shown that a specific form of inherited osteopetrosis in children is caused by a deficiency of carbonic anhydrase type II isoenzyme (Sly et al. 1985). These children also suffer from renal tubular acidosis due to a similar defect of proton sequence.

A genetic defect in the codon region for GM-CSF1 will result in the production of a defective protein by stromal cells in the osteoclast microenvironment and thus impair osteoclast formation. It has been shown that this disease can be cured by administration of exogenous GM-CSF1 (Felix et al. 1990). Moreover, expression of proto-oncogene src fos (Johnson et al. 1992) is also necessary for adequate osteoclast function (Soriano et al. 1991; Boyce et al. 1992a). C-src codes for a non-receptor tyrosine kinase which may be needed for the activation of the osteoclast. The essential substrate for this cytoplasmic kinase is unknown, although many of the proteins which are phosphorylated by this src-coded tyrosine kinase have been identified (Boyce et al. 1992b). An adequate "preparation" of the bone surface by release of mineral from the bone matrix appears to be required for normal bone resorption. This process seems to provide an optimal environment for maximal proteolytic activity of lysosomal enzymes released by the osteoclast, as well as for the activation of other factors released by immune cells and cells of the osteoblastic lineage. This paracrine effect acts directly on the osteoclasts and their precursors and controls the systemic endocrine effect of hormones on both bone resorption and calcium homeostasis. For the actual resorption process by mature multinucleated cells, attachment to the bone surface is also necessary. These adhesion molecules are integral cytoplasmic membrane proteins and bind to specific molecules in the bone matrix such as osteopontin and collagen types I and II. It is a common feature of these proteins that they contain specific Arg-Gly-Asp amino acid sequences. The binding process seems to be essential for bone resorption by osteoclasts, as synthetic peptide antagonists to Arg-Gly-Asp sequences could inhibit osteoclastic bone resorption in vitro (Sato et al. 1990). Furthermore, echistatin, which inhibits binding to the above-mentioned amino acid sequences, blocks bone resorption in vivo (Fisher et al. 1993).

References

Boyce BF, Yoneda T, Lowe C, et al (1992a) Requirement of pp60^{c-src} expression of osteoclasts to form ruffled borders and resorb bone. J Clin Invest 90:1622–1627

Boyce BF, Chen H, Bouton A, et al (1992b) A src tyrosine phosphoprotein substrate (P80/85) is localised to the ruffled border of osteoclasts in vitro. Br Dent J 156:216–220

Boyde A, Maconnachie E, Reid SA, et al (1986) Scanning electron microscopy in bone pathology: review of methods. Potential and application. Scanning Electron Microsc 4:1537–1554

Elion G, Mundy GR (1987) Direct resorption of bone by human breast cancer cells in vitro. Nature 276:726–728

Felix R, Cecchini MG, Fleisch H (1990) Macrophage colony stimulating factor restores in vivo bone resorption in the op/op osteopetrotic mouse. Endocrinology 127:92–94

Fisher JE, Caulfield MP, Sato M, et al (1993) Inhibition of osteoclastic bone resorption in vivo by echistatin, an arginyl-glycl-aspartyl (RGD)-containing protein. Endocrinology 132:1411–1413

Horton MA, Davies J (1989) Perspectives – adhesion receptors in bone. J Bone Miner Res 4:803–808

Johnson RS, Spiegelman BM, Papaloannou V (1992) Pleiotropic effects of a null mutation in the c-fos proto-oncogene. Cell 71:577–586

Jones SJ, Boyde A, Ali NN, et al (1985) A review of bone cell substratum interactions. Scanning 7:5–24

Kahn AJ, Stewart CC, Teitelbaum SL (1978) Contact-mediated bone resorption by human monocytes in vitro. Science 199:988–990

Mundy GR, Altman AJ, Gondek M, et al (1977) Direct resorption of bone by human monocytes. Science 196:1109–1111

Sato Y, Tsuboi R, Lyons R, et al (1990) Characterisation of the activation of latent TGFβ by co-cultures of endothelial cells and parasites or smooth muscle cells – a self-regulating system. J Cell Biol 111:757–763

Sly WS, Whyte MP, Sundaram V, et al (1985) Carbonic anhydrase II deficiency in 12 families with the autosomal recessive syndrome of osteopetrosis with renal tubular acidosis and cerebral calcification. N Engl J Med 313:139–145

Soriano P, Montgomery C, Geske R, et al (1991) Targeted disruption of the c-src proto-oncogene leads to osteopetrosis in mice. Cell 64:693–702

Bone Formation

Introduction

Bone formation is a more complex process than bone resorption. The formation process differs in the different sites of the skeleton: Endochondral bone formation takes place in the long bones and is characterized by an intermediate cartilage phase, whereas bone formation in the flat bones or at sites of previous resorption on endosteal surfaces and within the haversian systems occurs directly, without the cartilage phase. Fewer in vitro models have been developed to investigate bone formation than bone resorption.

Cells of the Osteoblast Lineage

The osteoblasts are derived from the stromal cell system. Fibroblasts, chondroblasts, reticular cells, and other bone-forming cells are also derived from the same stromal cell precursor (Owen 1985). The osteoblast family includes osteocytes and bone-lining cells covering the bone surface and the mature osteoblasts, which produce the proteins of the bone matrix, mainly collagen type I and osteocalcin. The later-mentioned peptide and the alkaline phosphatases and ectoenzymes produced by osteoblasts are frequently used as seromarkers of osteoblast and bone formation activity. Other products such as phospholipids and proteoglycans are also necessary for mineralization of the newly formed bone matrix. Osteoblasts are probably also required for physiological bone resorption, and they play an important role in bone remodeling. As described in the paragraphs on bone resorption, osteoblasts or their progenitor cells interact with osteoclasts or their precursors through paracrine function, through cell-to-cell contact, or by preparing the bone surface for attracting the osteoclast progenitors and for attachment of the mature osteoclast. Osteoblasts are also involved in the inhibition of bone resorption by bisphosphonates. They mediate the inhibitory effect through synthesis of an osteoclast resorption inhibitor (Kitté et al. 1995).

The major substance secreted by osteoblasts to form the bone matrix is collagen type I, which constitutes about 90% of the entire bone matrix. Post-translational modifications of collagen type I are specific for bone. These include hydroxylation of proline and lysine residues on collagen. The cross-linking occurs in the extracellular space and makes bone collagen type I very insoluble. The collagen molecules are packed end to end within the collagen fibril. Bone mineralization occurs when specific alignment of collagen molecules and other bone macromolecules such as fibronectin, osteonectin, and proteoglycans has occurred. The best-known of the diseases that are due to collagen type I disorders is osteogenesis imperfecta. Disorders of collagen type I production have also been implicated in osteoporosis, mainly through animal models. Heterozygotes of these animal models with osteogenesis imperfecta show the clinical phenotype of osteoporosis (Chipman et al. 1993). So far, the relationship between abnormalities of collagen type I and osteoporosis has not been proven. Osteonectin is the most frequently found noncollagen protein in the bone. It is secreted not only by osteoblasts but also by other mesenchymal cells. It is highly cross-linked and binds strongly to collagen type I and mineral surfaces such as hydroxyapatite. Its function is unknown.

Osteocalcin

Osteocalcin accounts for about 20% of the noncollagen proteins in the bone. It is most probably synthesized exclusively by osteoblasts in the presence of vitamin D_3. Osteocalcin contains 3-γ-carboxyglutamic acid residues that allow binding to calcium. This carboxylation is – as are many others in biology – vitamin K dependent. However, when this carboxylation was lacking because vitamin K activity had been blocked by warfarin, no osteocalcin was found in the skeleton in the rat model, but there were also no other detectable bone abnormalities (Price et al. 1982).

Other Bone Matrix Proteins

Other bone matrix proteins include fibronectin, osteopontin, and thrombospondin, as well as the bone sialoprotein and bone acidic glycoprotein. These proteins have a common Arg-Gly-Asp acid amino acid sequence and are responsible for mediating the attachment of these proteins to cell surfaces.

Bone Mineralization

One of the unique and important properties of bone is the mineralization of bone proteins. The mineral is deposited between the ends of two collagen molecules in a highly orderly way that does not cause disruption of the spatial orientation of the collagen fibril. Mineralization is carefully regulated at the nucleation site of the bone matrix rather than by simple precipitation, which would result in a random organization of the crystals. The initial site of mineral deposition appears to be the matrix vesicle. Extrusion of these vesicles occur at the cell surfaces next to the mineralizing bone. These vesicles are highly enriched with alkaline phosphatase and ATP, which prepare the bone matrix by removing inhibitors of mineralization. The process has been described in detail elsewhere (Posner 1987).

References

Chipman SD, Sweet HO, McBride DJ, et al (1993) Defective proalpha 2 (I) collagen synthesis in a recessive mutation in mice – a model of human osteogenesis imperfecta. Proc Natl Acad Sci U S A 90:7701–7705

Kitté C, Fleisch H, Günther HL (1995) Osteoblasts mediate the bisphosphonate inhibition on bone resorption through synthesis of an inhibitor of osteoclastic resorption. Bone 17:602 (abstract 18)

Owen M (1985) Lineage of osteogenic cells and their relationship to the stromal system. In: Peck WA (ed) Bone and mineral research, vol 3. Elsevier, New York, pp 1–26

Posner AS (1987) Bone mineral and the mineralization process. In: Peck WA (ed) Bone and mineral research, vol 5. Elsevier, New York, pp 65–116

Price PA, Williamson MK, Haba T, et al (1982) Excessive mineralization with growth plate closure in rats on chronic warfarin treatment. Proc Natl Acad Sci U S A 79:7734–7738

Factors Regulating Bone-resorbing Cells and Bone-forming Cells

Parathyroid Hormone

As previously mentioned, parathyroid hormone (PTH) is the most important factor for calcium homeostasis in the extracellular fluid. PTH plays a major role in bone resorption, but for the maintenance of the extracellular fluid calcium concentration its effect on the kidney is probably more important. The PTH effect on bone was described more than 50 years ago in patients with primary hyperparathyroidism (Albright et al. 1940) and than confirmed by autografting parathyroid glands to subcutaneous tissue over the calvariae of rats (Barnicot 1948). PTH – and PTH-related peptide (PTHrP) – is effective at concentrations of 10^{-9}–10^{-7} M. The rapid effect of PTH on bone resorption after a few hours' exposure (and the rapid response of the PTH to changes of ionized calcium concentration) suggests that PTH exerts its effect by activation of mature osteoclasts, whereas other factors such as vitamin D_3 exert their major effects on the recruitment and formation of osteoclasts. These findings lead to the hypothesis that PTH increases osteoclastic bone resorption when administered continuously but stimulates bone formation when administered intermittently in low doses.

This hypothesis is not supported by other data, however; mature osteoclasts do not have PTH receptors, although this observation made by most investigators is contradicted by other publications (Teti et al. 1991; Agarwala and Gay 1992). Probably, most PTH acts in the late osteoclast lineage directly or indirectly by production of other factors such as vitamin D_3 and interleukin-6 (Feyen et al. 1989). In vivo, other factors may contribute to the PTH effect. It has been shown that interleukin-1 (Stashenko et al. 1987) can enhance bone resorption and provoke hypercalcemia in vivo (Sabatini et al. 1988; Sato et al. 1989). Transforming growth factor a and epidermal growth factor can exert the same effect (Lorenzo and Quinton 1984; Yates et al. 1992).

Calcitonin

Calcitonin as PTH is a peptide hormone and is regulated by extracellular fluid calcium concentration. Its effect on calcium homeostasis is usually of short duration. It has therefore been hypothesized that calcitonin serves mainly to rapidly counteract calcium increase, e.g., associated with large calcium intake, associated with meals. The fact that calcitonin secretion is regulated by gastrointestinal hormones such as gastrin fits perfectly in the physiological model. Calcitonin receptors and inhibiting effects of calcitonin on bone resorption have been demonstrated at multiple levels in the osteoclast lineage (Kurihara et al. 1990). The effect of calcitonin on bone resorption is transient. The phenomenon of tachyphylaxis can also be seen when calcitonin is used in tumor-induced hypercalcemia. The loss of effectiveness can be inhibited by corticosteroids, at least in vitro (Wener et al. 1972), whereas most clinicians observe no beneficial effect of corticosteroids in tumor-induced hypercalcemia. However, these observations are contrary to those reported by others (Au 1975).

When calcitonin is used as a pharmacological agent in Paget's disease, tachyphylaxis is less commonly observed. The mechanism for this is unknown. Calcitonin is also used in the treatment of osteoporosis.

Life-threatening hypercalcemia is effectively controlled by concomitant administration of calcitonin and potent second- or third-generation bisphosphonates. The serum calcium level is more rapidly lowered by this combination than by bisphosphonates alone.

Vitamin D_3

The effect of vitamin D_3 on calcium homeostasis and bone remodeling has been described before. Vitamin D_3 deficiency due to low intake or malabsorption leads to impaired mineralization of the newly formed bone matrix; the disease is called osteomalacia. However, it has been known for many years that some metabolites of vitamin D are potent bone-resorbing factors (Raisz et al. 1972). Bone marrow mononuclear cells fuse to multinucleated cells with osteoclast characteristics when incubated with vitamin D_3. This phenomenon can also be seen in cells of the monocyte-macrophage lineage (Ibbotson et al. 1984; Roodman et al 1985). Vitamin D_3 probably does not act on mature osteoclasts, as no receptors are found in the mature nucleated cell and osteoclasts do not resorb bone in vitro unless cells of the osteoblast lineage are present. The model shows that vitamin D_3 exerts its effect rather as a differentiation agent on osteoclasts than through a direct influence on the mature osteoblast. This hypothesis is also supported clinically. In diseases in which osteoclasts fail to resorb bone, such as malignant osteopetrosis, vitamin D_3 can induce the appearance of active osteoclasts in bone sections and demonstrate bone resorption (Key et al. 1984).

Prostaglandins

The role of prostaglandins in the context of bone resorption is unclear, and contradicting observations have been made. The effects of prostaglandins may actually be bidirectional: short term with regard to bone inhibition and long term in the direction of bone resorption. Furthermore, species differences may be very important in determining the effects of prostaglandins on bone cell function, and sometimes opposite effects can be seen in different species. The results obtained in certain animal models are therefore not easily translated to other models or to human beings. Prostaglandins function also as mediators of other factors on bone resorption, such as epidermal growth factor and platelet-derived growth factor. The bone-resorbing effect of interleukin-1 can be partly inhibited by prostaglandin synthesis inhibitors such as indomethacin (Boyce et al. 1989).

Other metabolites of the arachidonic acid pathway, especially the leukotrienes, can also stimulate bone resorption (Meghji et al. 1988). Periarticular bone resorption in inflammatory diseases such as rheumatoid arthritis may be mediated by leukotrienes (Davidson et al. 1983).

Interleukin-1

Interleukin-1 (IL-1) is a potent stimulator of osteoclastic bone resorption. The effect is mediated at multiple sites in the osteoclast lineage. In osteopetrotic mice, who have nonfunctioning osteoclasts, the injection of IL-1 does not increase the ionized calcium compared with the respective wild-type mice. On the other hand, these osteopetrotic mice develop hypercalcemia when treated with PTH or PTH-rP because of the increased renal tubular calcium retention that is induced by these peptides. The regulatory effect of IL-1 is exerted by increased granulocyte-macrophage colony-forming unit activity (Uy et al. 1993), by induction of committed progenitor cell differentiation (Pfeilschifter et al. 1989), and perhaps also by direct activation of the mature osteoclast (Thomson et al. 1986). Both IL-1α and PTH-rP have been implicated in the pathogenesis of metastatic bone disease and hypercalcemia of solid tumors, as both factors are frequently produced in tumors which frequently develop bone metastases (Sato et al. 1989). On the other hand, IL-1β is produced by myeloma cells and acts as an autocrine growth factor of human myeloma cells through increased interleukin-6 production (Kawano et al. 1989); it has been linked to increased bone resorption in multiple myeloma. Increased production of IL-1β by circulating monocytes in the peripheral blood from patients with postmenopausal osteoporosis has been linked to the bone loss associated with this disease. The hypothesis is further supported by the observation that treatment with estrogens blocks the postmenopausal increase in blood monocyte IL-1 release (Pacifici et al. 1989)

The effects of IL-1α and -β on the interleukin receptors are blocked by the naturally occurring IL-1 receptor antagonist. It can inhibit hypercalcemia caused by IL-1α and -β in mice (Guise et al. 1987).

Tumor Necrosis Factor and Lymphotoxin

Both cytokines, tumor necrosis factor and lymphotoxin, share similar receptor mechanisms which seem to have identical effects on bone cells. Their effects on bone cells are also similar to those of IL-1. They also exert their effect at several steps in the macrophage-osteoclast lineage and mediate their effects at least partly through local production of prostaglandins. Lymphotoxin has been associated with hypercalcemia caused by malignant neoplasms of the lymphopoietic system such as lymphoma and myeloma (Garrett et al. 1987). Tumor necrosis factor also causes bone destruction and hypercalcemia of malignancy, although solid tumors usually do not produce tumor necrosis factor. However, some solid tumors can produce mediators such as GM-CSF, which then stimulate immune cells from the monocyte-macrophage lineage to produce tumor necrosis factor and cause hypercalcemia. Tumor necrosis factor has also been involved in bone destruction associated with chronic inflammatory diseases such as rheumatoid arthritis and in postmenopausal bone loss, since circulating monocytes from postmenopausal patients were found to produce an increased amount of tumor necrosis factor compared with monocytes from premenopausal controls or postmenopausal women with estrogen hormone replacement therapy.

Interleukin-4

Interkeukin-4 (IL-4) is a multifunctional cytokine which can inhibit bone resorption (Watanabe et al. 1990) in vitro. Osteoporosis has also been linked with IL-4 when mechanisms of bone loss were investigated in IL-4-transgenic mice (Lewis et al. 1992). IL-4 plays an important physiological and/or pathophysiological role that remains to be determined.

Interleukin-6

Interleukin-6 (IL-6) is a multifunctional cytokine which increases the formation of new osteoclasts from precursors. It increases also the number of multinucleated cells in human bone marrow cultures in combination with vitamin D_3 (Kurihara et al. 1990). The action of IL-6 with regard to bone resorption can be inhibited by neutralizing antibodies as well as by antisense oligonucleotides (Reddy et al 1993). IL-6 has been implicated in several types of bone remodeling disorders such as Paget's disease (Roodman et al. 1991) and postmenopausal bone loss (Jilka et al. 1992). IL-6 production by bone marrow-derived stromal cells and osteoblasts was inhibited by estradiol. This may be one of the potential mechanisms of the antiosteoporotic effect of estrogens (Girasole et al. 1992). IL-6 seems to play a major role as well in bone destruction and hypercalcemia associated with myeloma (Klein and Bataille 1991b). As previously described, IL-6 also serves as an autocrine growth factor in B-cell neoplasms such as myeloma. Increased IL-6 has been observed even in the peripheral blood of patients with plasma cell leukemia (Klein and Bataille 1991a, b).

γ-Interferon

γ-Interferon is a powerful inhibitor of both the formation and differentiation of osteoclasts. It seems more effective in inhibiting bone resorption mediated by IL-1 and tumor necrosis factor than the bone resorption stimulated by PTH or vitamin D_3 (Gowen and Mundy 1986). However, γ-interferon was not very useful in lowering serum calcium in vivo because of its toxicity (Klein and Bataille 1991 b).

Colony-stimulating Factors

Among the growth-regulatory factors of blood cells, the monocyte-macro-phage colony-stimulating factor (M-CSF) is important for the early steps of osteoclast recruitment (MacDonald et al. 1986). M-CSF does not stimulate bone resorption by activation of mature osteoclasts. The model is supported by the observation that in mice with a DNA coding defect in the region of M-CSF resulting in osteopetrosis, administration of M-CSF can cure the os-teoclastic function whereas transplantation of osteoclast precursors does not result in an improvement of osteoclast function (Felix et al. 1990). The ef-fects of GM-CSF have been described before.

Osteoclast-forming Factor

This peptide was only recently discovered and originates from a tumor which also produces GM-CSF, M-CSF, G-CSF, and IL-6 (Lee et al. 1991; Mun-dy 1995). The physiological and pathophysiological roles of this peptide remain to be determined.

References

Agarwala N, Gay CV (1992) Specific binding of parathyroid hormone on living osteoclasts. J Bone Miner Res 7:531–539

Albright F, Bloomberg F, Smith PH (1940) Postmenopausal osteoporosis. Trans Assoc Am Phys 55:298–305

Au WYW (1975) Calcitonin treatment of hypercalcemia due to parathyroid carcinoma: syn-ergistic effect of prednisone on long term treatment of hypercalcemia. Arch Intern Med 135:1594–1597

Barnicot NA (1948) The local effect of the parathyroid and other tissue on the bone in in-tracerebral grafts. J Anat 82:233–248

Boyce BF, Aufdemorte TB, Garrett IR, et al (1989) Effects of interleukin-1 on bone turnover in normal mice. Endocrinology 125:1142–1150

Davidson EM, Rae SA, Smith MJ (1983) Leukotriene B4, a mediator of inflammation pre-sent in synovial fluid in rheumatoid arthritis. Ann Rheum Dis 43:677–679

Felix R, Cecchini MG, Fleisch H (1990) Macrophage colony stimulating factor restores in vivo bone resorption in the op/op osteopetrotic mouse. Endocrinology 127:2592–2594

Feyen JHM, Elford P, Dipadova FE, et al (1989) Interleukin-6 is produced by bone and modulated by parathyroid hormone. J Bone Miner Res 4:633–638

Garrett IR, Durie BGM, Nedwin GE, et al (1987) Production of the bone resorbing cytokine lymphotoxin by cultured human myeloma cells. N Engl J Med 317:526–532

Girasole G, Jilka RL, Passaeri G, et al (1992) 17β-Estradiol inhibits interleukin-6 production by bone marrow derived stromal cells and osteoblasts in vitro. A potential mechanism for the antiosteoporotic effect of estrogens. J Clin Invest 89:883–891

Gowen M, Mundy GR (1986) Actions of recombinant interleukin-1, interleukin-2, and interferon gamma on bone resorption in vitro. J Immunol 136:2478–2482

Guise TA, Garrett IR, Bonewald LF, et al (1987) The interleukin-1 receptor antagonist inhibits hypercalcemia mediated by interleukin-1. J Bone Miner Res 8:583–588

Ibbotson KJ, Roodman GD, McManus LM, et al (1984) Identification and characterisation of osteoclast-like cells and their progenitors in cultures of feline marrow mononuclear cells. J Cell Biol 99:471–480

Jilka RL, Hangoc G, Girasole G, et al (1992) Increased osteoclast development after estrogen loss – mediation by interleukin-6. Science 257:88–91

Kawano M, Tanako H, Ishikawa H, et al (1989) Interleukin-1 accelerates autocrine growth of myeloma cells through interleukin-6 in human myeloma. Blood 73:2145–2148

Key L, Carnes D, Dole S, et al (1984) Treatment of congenital osteopetrosis with high dose calcitriol. N Engl J Med 310:410–415

Klein B, Bataille R (1991a) Recent advances in the biology of Il-6 in multiple myeloma. Cancer J 4:81–82

Klein B, Bataille R (1991b) Interleukin-6 in human multiple myeloma. M S Med Sci 7:937–943

Kurihara N, Bertolini D, Suda T, et al (1990) Interleukin-6 stimulates osteoclast-like multinucleated cell formation in long term human marrow cultures by including IL-1 release. J Immunol 144:426–430

Lee M, Eyre DR, Osborne WRA (1991) Isolation of a murine osteoclast colony-stimulating factor. Proc Natl Acad Sci U S A 88:8500–8504

Lewis DB, Liggit D, Teitelbaum S, et al (1992) Mechanism of osteoporosis in IL-4 transgenic mice. J Bone Miner Res 7 [Suppl 1]:20

Lorenzo JA, Quinton J (1984) Epidermal growth factor enhances the resorptive response to parathyroid hormone. Calcif Tissue Int 36:465

MacDonald BR, Mundy GR, Clark S, et al (1986) Effects of human recombinant CSF-GM and highly purified CSF-1 on the formation of multinucleated cells with osteoclast characteristics in long term bone marrow cultures. J Bone Miner Res 1:227–233

Meghji S, Sandy JR, Scutt AM, et al (1988) Stimulation of bone resorption by lipoxygenase metabolites of arachidonic acid. Prostaglandins 36:139–147

Mundy GR (1995) Factor regulating bone resorbing and born forming cells in bone remodeling and its disorders. Martin Dunitz, London, p 55

Pacifici R, Rifas L, McCracken R, et al (1989) Ovarian steroid treatment blocks a postmenopausal increase in blood monocyte interleukin-1 release. Proc Natl Acad Sci USA 86:2398–2402

Pfeilschifter J, Chenu C, Bird A, et al (1989) Interleukin-1 and tumor necrosis factor stimulate the formation of human osteoclast-like cells in vitro. J Bone Miner Res 4:113–118

Raisz LG, Trummel CL, Holick MF, et al (1972) 1,25-Dihydroxycholecalciferol: a potent stimulator of bone resorption in tissue culture. Science 175:768–769

Reddy SV, Neckars L, Dallas M, et al (1993) Antisense constructs to IL-6 mRNA inhibit bone resorption by osteoclasts (OCL) from giant cell tumors (GCT) of bone. Clin Res 41:184A

Roodman GD, Ibbotson KJ, MacDonald BR, et al (1985) 1,25-Dihydroxyvitamin D_3 causes formation of multinucleated cells with several osteoclast characteristics in cultures of primate marrow. Proc Natl Acad Sci U S A 82:8213–8217

Roodman GD, Kurihara N, Ohsaki Y, et al (1991) Interleukin-6 a potential autocrine/paracrine factor in Paget's disease of bone. J Clin Invest 89:46–52

Sabatini M, Boyce B, Aufdemorte T, et al (1988) Infusions of recombinant human interleukin-1α and β cause hypercalcemia in normal mice. Proc Natl Acad Sci U S A 85:5235–5239

Sato K, Fujii Y, Kasono K, et al (1989) Parathyroid hormone-related protein and interleukin-1α synergistically stimulate bone resorption in vitro and increase the serum calcium concentration in mice in vivo. Endocrinology 124:2172–2138

Stashenko P, Dewhrist FE, Peros WJ, et al (1987) Synergistic interactions between interleukin-1, tumor necrosis factor, and lymphotoxin in bone resorption. J Immunol 138:1464–1468

Teti A, Rizzoli R, Zambonin-Zallone A (1991) Parathyroid hormone binding to cultured avian osteoclasts. Biochem Biophys Res Commun 174:1217–1222

Thomson BM, Saklatvala J, Chambers TJ (1986) Osteoblasts mediate interleukin-1 stimulation of bone resorption by rat osteoclast. J Exp Med 164:104–112

Uy HL, Dallas M, Wright K, et al (1993) Multipotent hematopoietic osteoclast precursors are increased by interleukin-1 in vivo. J Bone Miner Res 8:1084

Watanabe K, Tanaka Y, Morimoto I, et al (1990) Interleukin-4 as a potent inhibitor of bone resorption. Biochem Biophys Res Commun 172:1035–1041

Wener JA, Gorton SJ, Raisz LG (1972) Escape from inhibition of resorption in cultures of fetal bone treated with calcitonin and parathyroid hormone. Endocrinology 90:752–759

Yates AJP, Favarato G, Aufdemorte TB, et al (1992) Expression of human transforming growth factor a by Chinese hamster ovarian tumors in nude mice causes hypercalcemia and increased osteoclastic bone resorption. J Bone Miner Res 7:847–853

Factors Regulating Bone Formation

The proteins described in the previous paragraph are not only structural proteins; they can also have regulatory effects on bone formation. Other proteins in the bone matrix are even more powerful and appear to modulate bone formation by a paracrine pathway on the osteoblast lineage. They hold the position of linkage in the bone remodeling model between bone resorption and formation, as well as in bone repair of fractures.

Transforming Growth Factor β (TGF-β)

TGF-β is the most powerful promoter of bone formation (Noda and Camiliere 1989). It is present in bone as a latent complex in several forms, for instance, bound to β-2 macroglobulin. All these latent forms can be activated by exposure to acid. The acidic microenvironment under the osteoclast is an ideal site for activation of TGF-β. This activation can happen directly or be induced by proteolytic enzymes. TGF-β not only activates osteoblasts but also increases the capacity of the latter to migrate unidirectionally (Pfeilschifter et al. 1989). TGF-β also has effects on the osteoclasts which can be partially inhibited by indomethacin, suggesting that at least parts of these effects on osteoclasts are mediated by prostaglandins of the E-series (Pfeilschifter et al. 1988).

Fibroblast Growth Factors

Fibroblast growth factors may exert their effects on bone formation indirectly, since it was found that they enhance TGF-β expression (Rodan et al. 1989).

Platelet-derived Growth Factor

Platelet-derived growth factor stimulates osteoblast proliferation and is produced by cells with an osteoblast phenotype, including osteosarcoma cells. It may act as an autocrine growth factor, as these cells also contain receptors for it (Graves et al. 1983, 1984). Platelet-derived growth factor may also regulate bone resorption, but results from animal models are contradictory, as this observation was made only in mice (Tashjian et al. 1982) but not in rats. Platelet-derived growth factor may be also involved in the model of bone remodeling, acting as a coupling factor there by linking bone formation with previous bone resorption.

Bone Morphogenetic Proteins

These peptides have sequence homology with TGF-β but different effects. They enhance the differentiating function of osteoblasts (Harris et al. 1992). They have the unique ability to stimulate the formation of ectopic bone when injected intramuscularly or subcutaneously (Urist 1965). Their role in the bone remodeling process is yet to be determined. However, these proteins have been shown to be extremely effective in enhancing repair of segmental bone defects. They may have implications for fracture healing (Rozen 1993).

Insulin-like Growth Factors

Insulin-like growth factors (IGF) are important for the mediation of growth hormone effects on bone cells (Canalis 1980). Transient exposure of PTH can also lead to enhanced production of IGF-1 in organ cultures (Canalis et al. 1989). IGF-2 is also present in the bone matrix and acts as a skeletal growth factor (Mohan et al. 1988). Again, both IGF-1 and IGF-2 have been linked with the proposed coupling mechanism of osteoblastic and osteoclastic bone remodeling.

References

Canalis E (1980) Effect of insulin-like growth factor I on DNA and protein synthesis in cultured fetal rat calvaria. J Clin Invest 66:709–719

Canalis E, Centrella M, Burch W, et al (1989) Insulin-like growth factor-1 mediates selective anabolic effects of parathyroid hormone in bone cultures. J Clin Invest 83:60–65

Graves DT, Owen AJ, Antoniades HN (1983) Evidence that a human osteosarcoma cell line which secretes a mitogen similar to platelet-derived growth factor requires growth factors present in platelet-poor plasma. Cancer Res 43:83–87

Graves DT, Owen AJ, Barth RK, et al (1984) Detection of c-sis transcripts and synthesis of PDGF-like proteins by human osteosarcoma cells. Science 226:972–974

Harris SE, Harris MA, Feng JW, et al (1992) Expression of bone morphogenetic proteins (BMPs) during differentiation of fetal rat calvarial osteoblasts in vitro. J Bone Miner Res 7:12

Mohan S, Jennings TA, Linkhardt JE, et al (1988) Primary structure of human skeletal growth factor (SGF): homology with IGF-2. J Bone Miner Res 3:598

Noda M, Camiliere JJ (1989) In vivo stimulation of bone formation by transforming growth factor β. Endocrinology 124:2991–2994

Pfeilschifter J, Wolf O, Naumann A, et al (1989) Chemotactic response of osteoblast-like cells to transforming growth factor β. J Bone Miner Res 5:825–830

Pfeilschifter JP, Seyedin S, Mundy GR (1988) Transforming growth factor β inhibits bone resorption in fetal rat long bone cultures. J Clin Invest 82:680–685

Rodan SB, Wesolowski G, Thomas KA, et al (1989) Effects of acidic and basic fibroblast growth factors on osteoblastic cells. Connect Tissue Res 20:283–288

Rozen V (1993) Bone morphogenetic proteins. In: Mundy GR, Martin TJ (eds) Physiology and pharmacology of bone. Springer, Berlin Heidelberg New York, pp 725–748

Tashjian AH, Hohmann EL, Antoniades HN, et al (1982) Platelet-derived growth factor stimulates bone resorption via a prostaglandin mediated mechanism. Endocrinology 111:118–124

Urist MR (1965) Bone: formation by autoinduction. Science 150:893

Pharmacological Treatment of Bone Disorders

The pharmacological approach to disorders of bone remodeling is based mainly on drugs that inhibit osteoclastic bone resorption. Fewer advances have been made in the development of drugs to stimulate bone formation.

Estrogens and Antiestrogens

At sufficient dosages, all estrogens are effective inhibitors of rapid bone loss during the postmenopausal period. This seems to be the only area where there is little controversy. The question of estrogen therapy in established osteoporosis provokes more discussion than the question of prevention. Hormone replacement therapy in the young postmenopausal patient population has been shown to protect against rapid bone loss and the risk of later development of osteoporotic fractures (Weiss et al. 1980). This has been confirmed by other investigators (Ettinger et al. 1985).

As previously described, estrogens inhibit the activation of osteoclasts on bone-resorbing surfaces (Parfitt 1979). The roles of IL-1 and IL-6 have been discussed in the preceding chapter. However, estrogens do not inhibit all forms of osteoclastic bone resorption. They are not effective in the treatment of tumor-induced hypercalcemia or Paget's disease. The estrogen receptor content of bone cells is low (Erikssen et al. 1988; Oursler et al. 1991). The effect of estrogens may be mediated by modulation of factors released by osteoblasts, which influence osteoclast activity in a paracrine fashion. The mechanism by which estrogens inhibit bone resorption remains unknown so far. Tamoxifen, a non-steroidal antiestrogen is established as the endocrine therapy of choice, in breast cancer both in advanced disease and in the adjuvant setting. The differential actions of tamoxifen occur by selective estrogen-receptor modulation at different target sites to produce estrogenic or antiestrogenic effect. Long-term administration of tamoxifen produces estrogen-like effects that maintain bone-density and lower circulating low density lipoprotein cholesterol (Powles et al. 1990; Powles et al. 1996; Bilimoria et al. 1996). The influence of tamoxifen on the incidence of clinical relevant fracture rates in breast cancer patients is much less clear. Recently available data from an American breast cancer prevention study (NSABP-P1) in healthy women at increased risk to develop breast cancer showed that fractures in the tamoxifen-treated group occur less frequent than in the placebo-treated group (Wickerham et al. 1998).

New antiestrogen-analogues maintaining the beneficial effect on bone and lipids, but lacking the stimulatory effects in the uterus have been developed. Toremifen (Grams et al. 1998), droloxifen (Ke et al. 1995) and idoxifene (Coombes et al. 1995) have been developed as anticancer agents whereas raloxifen – developed as antiosteoporotic agent – has not only been shown to inhibit the osteoporotic process (Delmas et al. 1997) but has also proved to decrease the incidence of breast cancer to one third as compared to women in the placebo group in the two-year findings from the MORE trial (Jordan et al. 1998).

Calcium

Oral calcium has been widely used in the prevention and treatment of osteoporosis. Negative calcium balance associated with low calcium intake is present in many osteoporosis patients (Heaney et al. 1982). It is widely accepted that early, sufficient calcium intake is necessary to maintain an adequate calcium balance. This ensures normal bone growth. Calcium-deficient nutrition habits can aggravate bone loss associated with menopause (Heany 1991; Johnston et al. 1992). However, the role of oral calcium therapy in the treatment of established osteoporosis is still controversial. Additional studies have raised questions rather than given answers and explanations. Although it was shown that people with low calcium intake have an increased incidence of hip fractures in later life (Matkovic et al. 1979), more recent studies have shown that this increased risk of hip fracture with low calcium intake may not be relevant unless the daily calcium intake falls below 100 mg/day (Lau et al. 1988). Physical activity and possibly other lifestyle parameters (and probably the use of estrogen) may also influence the hip fracture rate among the aging population (Cooper et al. 1988). Oral calcium therapy is supposed to suppress PTH secretion and to increase calcitonin secretion in patients with osteoporosis (Riggs et al. 1976). This leads to an improvement in calcium balance, which is presumably beneficial. Sufficient calcium intake seems most important in adolescent girls, as this segment of the population is the most deficient in dietary calcium at the time when oral calcium may be important for the development of peak bone mass. Negative calcium balance can also be corrected in postmenopausal patients, but this cannot replace estrogen therapy in order to reduce accelerated bone loss. It is reasonable to restore calcium balance with 1000 mg elemental calcium daily for teenagers and 1500 mg daily for postmenopausal women. Calcium carbonate is most widely used, but the calcium citrate is an alternative, particularly for elderly women who may be achlorhydric, since the bioavailability of the citrate is better.

Fluoride

Fluoride has also been used in postmenopausal osteoporosis for many years and has remained a controversial issue for many reasons, for instance, insufficient efficacy and concern regarding side effects such as the risk of increased bone fragility (Riggs et al. 1990). Supporters of fluoride therapy criticize these studies as having used doses that were too high and end points of minor relevance, such as radiological abnormalities rather than clinically important factors, and as therefore being inconclusive. Fluoride therapy increases trabecular bone formation. Fluoride may act directly on bone cells, thus inhibiting the activity of osteoblast acid phosphatase, which is responsible for the dephosphorylation of tyrosine kinases (Farley et al. 1983; Lau et al. 1989). This effect leads to enhanced tyrosine kinase activity and potentially enhances the effects of growth factors. The newly formed bone is structurally abnormal, with mineralization defects, but the effect is associated with high doses of fluoride only. If oral calcium and vitamin D are supplemented, this mineralization defect does not occur. Fluoride therapy increases the bone mass in about 70% of osteoporotic patients by 10% per year, as measured by bone mineral density. Obviously, fluoride therapy is theoretically indicated for patients with low-turnover osteoporosis. The most effective dose is probably in the range of 60–75 mg sodium fluoride (NaF) daily, although beneficial effects may be seen with 30 mg NaF daily. However, the therapeutic window is narrow. Maximal effects are reached with serum concentrations of 10 µmol/l, whereas 15 µmol/l may be toxic. The importance of bioavailability of the preparations with special regard to the narrow therapeutic window has been discussed elsewhere (Nagant et al. 1990).

Vitamin D$_3$/Calcitriol

Calcitriol (1,25-dihydroxyvitamin D$_3$) is the most widely used preparation of the active vitamin D metabolite in the pharmacological treatment of disorders of bone remodeling. This fat-soluble vitamin is well absorbed by the gastrointestinal tract in individuals with normal intestinal absorption. It increases calcium absorption from the gut, promotes normal mineralization of the bone, and decreases PTH secretion. The efficacy of the vitamin D metabolite is variable. In renal bone disease it clearly decreases PTH secretion and promotes normal mineralization of the bone, whereas it does not correct the mineralization defect associated with aluminum toxicity. Its efficacy in osteoporosis is still under debate; reports in the literature are contradictory. Some studies found an increase in bone mass and a decrease of vertebral fractures (Lindholm et al. 1982; Orimo et al. 1987) and hip fractures (Chapuy et al. 1992). Others have shown decreased bone mass and increased fracture rate (Ott and Chesnut 1989; Finn et al. 1982). In the United States and Europe calcitriol is generally used in a dose of 0.25 µg/day in patients with low-turnover osteoporosis who have low calcium intake due to either dietary conditions or low absorption from the gut and low calcitriol concentration in the serum. Urinary calcium excretion is usually below 100 mg/24 h. Other vitamin D metabolites, such as ergocalciferol (vitamin D_2) in doses of 1–10 mg/day and dihydrotachysterol in a dose of 0.1–1 mg/day, can also be used. The latter is used mainly in Japan.

Phosphate Therapy

Oral phosphate therapy is used in primary hyperparathyroidism where serum phosphate is low. It has been used in the past in the treatment of tumor-induced hypercalcemia. It binds calcium in the gut and decreases its absorption and inhibits osteoclastic bone resorption (Yates et al. 1991). Oral phosphate therapy is almost always effective in patients with primary hyperparathyroidism, at least transiently (Mundy et al. 1983). It can also be used in tumor-induced hypercalcemia, but it is not the treatment of choice and has to be used with caution as it frequently leads to soft tissue calcium deposition, especially when given rapidly to patients with moderate to severe hypercalcemia who have poor renal function and high serum phosphate levels (Carey et al. 1968). Furthermore, visceral damage with acute renal failure (Ayala et al. 1975) and damage to other organ sites (Dudly and Blackburn 1970) have been reported.

Further treatments for hypercalcemia and malignant osteolytic bone disease are described below.

References

Ayala G, Chertow BS, Shah JH, et al (1975) Acute hyperphosphataemia and acute persistent renal insufficiency induced by oral phosphate therapy. Ann Intern Med 83:520–521

Bilimoria MM, Assikis VJ, Jordan VD (1996) Should adjuvant tamoxifen therapy be stopped at 5 years? Cancer J Sci Am 2:140–150

Carey RW, Schmitt GW, Kobald HH (1968) Massive extraskeletal calcification during phosphate treatment of hypercalcemia. Arch Intern Med 122:150–155

Chapuy MC, Arlot ME, Duboeuf, et al (1992) Vitamin D_3 and calcium to prevent hip fractures in the elderly woman. N Engl J Med 327:1637–1642

Coombes RC, Haynes BC, Dousett M, Quigley M, English J, Judson IR, Griffs LJ, Potter GA, McCaque R, Jarman M (1995) Idoxifene: Report of a phase I study with patients with metastatic breast cancer. Cancer Res 55:1070–1074

Cooper C, Barker DJP, Wickham C (1988) Physical activity, muscle strength and calcium intake and fracture of the proximal femur in Britain. Br Med J 297:1443–1446

Cummings SR, Norton L, Eckert S, Grady D, Kauley J, Knickerbocker R, Black D, Nickelson T, Glusman J, Krueger K (for the MORE investigators 1998) Raloxifen reduces the risk of breast cancer and may decrease the risk of endometrial cancer in post-menopausal women. Two-year findings from the multiple outcomes of raloxifen evaluation (MORE) trial. Proc Am Soc Slin Oncol 17:3

Delmas PD, Bjarnason NH, Mitlak BH, Ravoux AC, Shan AS, Huster WJ, Draper M, Christiansen C (1997) Effects of raloxifene on bone mineral mensity, srum cholesterol concentrations, and uterine endometrium in postmenopausal women. New Engl J Med 4, 337:1641–1647

Dudly FJ, Blackburn CRB (1970) Extraskeletal calcification complicating oral neurophosphate therapy. Lancet 2:628–630

Erikssen EF, Colvard DS, Berg NJ (1988) Evidence of estrogen receptors in normal human osteoblast-like cells. Science 241:84–86

Ettinger B, Genant HK, Cann CE (1985) Long-term estrogen replacement therapy prevents bone loss and fractures. Ann Intern Med 102:319–324

Farley JR, Wergedal JE, Baylink DJ (1983) Fluoride directly stimulates proliferation and alkaline phosphatase activity of bone-formation cells. Science 222:330–332

Finn GF, Christiansen C, Transbol I (1982) Treatment of postmenopausal osteoporosis. A controlled therapeutic trial comparing oestrogen/gestagen, 1,25-dihydroxyvitamin D, and calcium. Clin Endocrinol (Oxf) 16:515–524

Gams R, Sasco AJ, Smith LL, Powles TJ, Toninaga T, Holli K (1998) Fareston – a new choice in anto-oestrogen therapy. Eur J Cancer, in press

Heany RP (1991) Life-long calcium intake and prevention of bone fragility in the aged. Calcif Tissue Int 49:S42–S45

Heaney RP, Gallagher JC, Johnston CC, et al (1982) Calcium nutrition and bone health in the elderly. Am J Clin Nutr 36:986–1013

Johnston CC Jr, Miller JZ, Slemenda CW, et al (1992) Calcium supplement and increases in bone mineral density in children. N Engl J Med 327:82–87

Jordan V, Glusman J, Eckert S, Lippmann M, Powles T, Costa A, Morrow M, Norton L (1998) Incident primary breast cancer are reduced by raloxifene: integrated data from multicenter, double-blind, randomized trials in ≈ 12,000 postmenopausal women. Proc Am Soc Clin Oncol 17:122a

Ke HZ, Chen HK, Simmons HA, Pirie CM, Ma YF, Jee WSS, Thompson DD (1995) Droloxifen, a new estrogen agonist, prevents ovariectomy-induces bone loss in growing and aged female rats. Endocrinology 136:2435–2441

Lau E, Donnan S, Barker DJP, et al (1988) Physical activity and calcium intake in fracture of the proximal femur in Hong Kong. Br Med J 297:1441–1443

Lau KH, Farley JR, Freeman TK, et al (1989) A proposed mechanism of the mitogenic action of fluoride on bone cells: inhibition of the activity of an osteoblastic acid phosphatase. Metabolism 38:858–868

Lindholm TS, Nilsson OS, Widhe T, et al (1982) Preventive treatment of osteoporosis with 1-alpha-hydroxyvitamin D_3 and calcium. Evaluation of bone histomorphometry in osteoporotic and age matched controls. Acta Vitaminol Enzymol 4:179–184

Matkovic V, Kostial K, Simonovic I, et al (1979) Bone status and fracture rates in two regions of Yugoslavia. Am J Clin Nutr 32:540–549

Mundy GR, Wilkinson R, Heath DA (1983) Comparative study of available medical therapy for hypercalcemia of malignancy. Am J Med 74:421–432

Nagant C, Devogelaer JP, Stein F (1990) Fluoride treatment for osteoporosis. Lancet 336:48–49

Orimo H, Shiraki M, Hayashi T, et al (1987) Reduced occurrence of vertebral crush fractures in senile osteoporosis treated with 1-alpha-(OH)-vitamin D_3. Bone Miner 3:1916–1919

Ott SM, Chesnut CH III (1989) Calcitriol treatment is not effective in postmenopausal osteoporosis. Ann Intern Med 110:267–274

Oursler MJ, Osdoby P, Pyfferson J, et al (1991) Avian osteoclasts as estrogen target cells. Proc Natl Acad Sci U S A 88:6613–6617

Parfitt AM (1979) Quantum concept of bone remodeling and turnover: implications for the pathogenesis of osteoporosis. Calcif Tissue Int 28:1–5

Powles T, Tillyer C, Jones A, Ashley S, Treleaven J, Davey J, McKima J (1990) Prevention of breast cancer with tamoxifen – an update on the Royal Marsden Hospital pilot programme. Eur J Cancer 26:680–684

Powles, Hickish T, Kanis JA, Tidy A, Ashley S (1996) Effect of tamoxifen on bone mineral density measured by dual-energy X ray absorptometry in healthy premenopausal and postmenopausal women. J Clin Oncol 14:78–84

Riggs BL, Jowsey J, Kelly PJ, et al (1976) Effects of oral therapy with calcium and vitamin D in primary osteoporosis. J Clin Endocrinol Metab 42:1139–1144

Riggs BL, Hodgson SF, O'Fallon WM, et al (1990) Effect of fluoride treatment on the fracture rate in postmenopausal women with osteoporosis. N Engl J Med 322:802–809

Yates AJP, Oreffo ROC, Mayor K, et al (1991) Inhibition of bone resorption by inorganic phosphate is mediated both by reduced osteoclast formation and by impaired activity of mature osteoclasts. J Bone Miner Res 6:437–438

Weiss NS, Ure CL, Ballard JH, et al (1980) Decreased risk of fractures of the hip and lower forearm with postmenopausal use of estrogen. N Engl J Med 303:1195–1198

Wickerham DL, Costantino JC, Fisher B, Kavanah M, Cronin W, Vogel V, Robidoux A, Daly M, Ford L, Redmond CK, Wolmark N (1998) The initial results from NSABP Protocol P-1: A clinical trial to determine the worth of tamoxifen for preventing breast cancer in women at increased risk. Proc Am Soc Clin Oncol 17:3a

Bisphosphonates

Pamidronate: From a Detergent in Washing Powder to a Registered Drug

The first bisphosphonate was synthesized more than 100 years ago – in 1897 – by von Beyer and Hoffmann. Sixty-three years elapsed before they were cited again by Blazer and Worms of Henkel and Co. GmbH as complexing agents in alkaline solution for bivalent ions such as calcium and magnesium. Henkel intended to use these compounds, which were then still called diphosphonates, not only as an additive in washing powder but also in cosmetics and other products such as toothpaste. The state authorities then required a "minipharmacology" with special regard to toxicology. One of the members of the board of directors of Henkel at that time was also on the executive board of the Ciba company. This was the Ciba's first contact with bisphosphonates. At that time, Ciba still had no official interest in the bisphosphonates, but Prof. Hobitz, a radiopharmacologist who came from Geigy after the two companies merged, was informed because he was busy investigating questions regarding calcium metabolism. Voltaren® (diclofenac sodium) and calcitonin were developed in his unit. He decided to follow the development of the then-called diphosphonates as a side project. Finally, a 5-year option on a patent for a second-generation compound, pamidronate, was obtained from Henkel, only for endocrine indications (Mühlemann et al. 1970). At the same time, Olaf Bijvoet from the Metabolic Unit of the University of Leiden also consulted Henkel GmbH for pharmacologic/toxicologic purposes with the intention of using these compounds in toothpaste and selling them for medical indications. Prof. Bijvoet investigated many bisphosphonates manufactured by Henkel and finally started to use such compounds as medical drugs. The pamidronate produced by Henkel was not completely stable and therefore not very useful for research in the medical field. Ciba developed this compound further and initiated new toxicologic and pharmacologic investigations. The story would be rather incomplete without mention of Prof. Herbert Fleisch from the Department of

Pathophysiology of the University of Berne, who began studies with inorganic pyrophosphate in 1960. He investigated the question: "Why do not all collagenous tissues mineralize?", as collagen with nucleating activity had been extracted from both mineralizing and nonmineralizing tissues. He thus examined the possibility that inhibitors of calcification might exist which would be destroyed locally at the site of mineralization and found that plasma indeed contained inhibitory activity against calcium phosphate precipitation and that part of this activity could be destroyed by alkaline phosphatase (Fleisch und Neuman 1961). (Pyro)phosphate had been known for a long time – since 1940, to inhibit precipitation of calcium carbonate (Bührer und Reitemeyer 1940; Reitemeyer und Bührer 1940). Further investigations showed that pyrophosphates were very powerful inhibitors of calcium phosphate precipitation at concentrations as low as 10^{-6} M. These compounds were found in many biological fluids and inhibited both crystal aggregation and crystal solution of calcium phosphate. Later, in collaboration with S. Bisatz, Prof. Fleisch was able to verify the above-mentioned hypothesis. He also found inhibitory activity in urine, in much higher amounts than in plasma. They isolated one of the inhibitors, which proved to be inorganic pyrophosphate (Fleisch and Bisatz 1962). This observation suggested that it might be a compound of physiological and pathophysiological significance, perhaps in hyperphosphatasia and in renal lithiasis. Unfortunately, pyrophosphate is rapidly degraded in vivo and is therefore not useful as a medical drug.

Prof. Fleisch and co-workers later showed that pyrophosphate not only inhibited crystallization of calcium phosphate from solutation but also slowed the transformation of amorphous calcium phosphate to its crystallized form (Fleisch et al. 1968 a). Further investigations suggested that pyrophosphate might have both physiological and pathophysiological significance as it might protect soft tissues from mineralization (Fleisch et al. 1965). Pyrophosphate has been linked to calcium oxalate precipitation and its relation to urolithiasis (Fleisch and Bisatz 1964; Fleisch et al. 1964). In 1966, Prof. Fleisch was invited to give a lecture at the Procter and Gamble Company in Cincinnati, Ohio, USA. This company had had a long-standing interest in the dental field and had investigated several analogues of pyrophosphate, the then-called diphosphonates, in order to develop topical agents for use against dental calculus. Ethane-1-hydroxy-1,1-disphosphonate (etidronate) was found to be a powerful inhibitor of calcium phosphate crystallization. This visit in Cincinnati led to the collaboration of Prof. Fleisch's unit and Procter and Gamble. Their work confirmed that the diphosphonates had physical and chemical effects similar to those of pyrophosphate. They also inhibited calcium phosphate dissolution. The first biological effect reported was the ability of the compounds to prevent ectopic calcification. In addition, and in contrast to pyrophosphate, they also inhibited bone resorption (Fleisch et al. 1968 b, 1969). The way to their clinical use was set.

Like most other bisphosphonates, pamidronate also went through the laboratory of Prof. Fleisch, who generated the important preclinical data for the further development of this drug. Later, pamidronate came into the clinics of several investigators who were developing pamidronate in collaboration with Ciba. Early studies were done in the Rheumatology Department of the University of Basel (Prof. Müller) and in the Department of Internal Medicine of the University Hospital in Lausanne (Prof. Burckardt). Most of the pharmacokinetic data which finally served for registration purposes with the state authorities were obtained in the United Kingdom. Clinically, pamidronate has been used in Paget's disease and tumor-induced hypercalcemia. Its application in some other rare conditions such as bone lesions in Gaucher's disease (Samuel et al. 1994) and impaired fracture healing in the Kasabach-Merritt syndrome (Korte W, Thürlimann B, Blatter G, unpublished data) has been investigated with success. Many phase-II studies evaluating various end points in malignant osteolytic bone disease were later undertaken. Systematic dose-escalation studies and randomized placebo-controlled trials were conducted in the early 1990s and led to registration of the drug for this indication. Currently under investigation are the treatment of osteoporosis, its prevention, and bone loss associated with corticosteroids and hematological diseases. Further trials of pamidronate as an adjuvant treatment in breast cancer are also ongoing.

References

Bührer T, Reitemeyer R (1940) The inhibiting action of minute amounts of sodium hexamethaphosphate on the precipitation of calcium carbonate from ammoniacal solutions. J Phys Chem 1944:552–574

Fleisch H, Bisatz S (1962) Mechanism of calcification: inhibitory role of pyrophosphate. Nature 195:911

Fleisch H, Bisatz S (1964) The inhibitory effect of pyrophosphate on calcium oxalate precipitation and its relation to urolithiasis. Experimenta 20:276

Fleisch H, Neuman WF (1961) Mechanisms of calcification: role of collagen polyphosphate and phosphatase. Am J Physiol 200:1296–1300

Fleisch H, Bisatz S, Care AD (1964) Effect of orthophosphate on urinary pyrophosphate excretion and the prevention of urolithiasis. Lancet 1:1065–1067

Fleisch H, Schibler D, Maerki J, Frossard I (1965) Inhibition of aortic calcification by means of pyrophosphates and polyphosphates. Nature 207:1300–1301

Fleisch H, Rossell RGG, Bisatz S, Termine JD, Bosner AS (1968a) Influence of pyrophosphate on the transformation of amorphous to crystalline calcium phosphate. Calcif Tissue Res 2:49–59

Fleisch H, Roussell RGG, Bisatz S, Casey PA Mühlbauer R (1968b) The influence of pyrophosphate analogues (diphosphonates) on the precipitation and dissolution of calcium phosphate in vitro and in vivo. Calcif Tissue Res 2:10A

Fleisch H, Roussell RGG, Francis ND (1969) Diphosphonates inhibit hydroxyapatite dissolution in vitro and bone resorption in tissue cultures and in vivo. Science 165:1262–1264

Mühlemann HR, Bobler D, Schatt A, Berni Moulin JP (1970) Effect of bisphosphonate on human supragingival calculus. Helv Odont Acta 14:31

Reitemeyer R, Bührer T (1940) The inhibiting action of minute amounts of sodium hexamethaphosphate on the precipitation of calcium carbonate from ammoniacal solutions. J Phys Chem 1944:535–551

Samuel R, Katz K, Papadopoulos SE, Yosipovitch Z, Zaizov R, Liberman UA (1994) APD treatment improves the clinical skeletal manifestations of Gaucher's disease. Pediatrics 94:385–389

Chemical Structure and Preclinical Evaluation

Chemical Structure

Bisphosphonates are derivatives of pyrophosphate. The characteristic P-O-P structure of pyrophosphate has been replaced by a P-C-P structure. A great variation is possible by changing the two lateral chains on the carbon atom or by esterifying the phosphate groups. Thousands of bisphosphonates have been synthesized and many tested. Alendronate, clodronate, etidronate, ibandronate, pamidronate, and tiludronate are commercially available in some countries. Some relationship of their structure to the spectrum of biological effects has been observed. Many of the analogues have properties similar to those of pyrophosphate but, unlike pyrophosphate, the P-C-P core structure has made them completely resistant to enzymatic degradation. Bisphosphonates are stable to heat and to most chemical agents. Each molecule has its own physical, chemical, and biological characteristics according to their side chains, although these P-C-P compounds have many common properties. It is impossible to extrapolate with certainty from the data of one compound to other bisphosphonates. The chemical structure of the bisphosphonates used in human beings can be seen in Fig. 1 (from H. Fleisch).

Biological Effects

Many in vitro and in vivo models have been developed to investigate the actions of bisphosphonates. These are described elsewhere and are reviewed by H. Fleisch, who has more than 25 years' experience in the preclinical development of bisphosphonates. Virtually all bisphosphonates "went through his institution" before being further developed by pharmaceutical companies and clinicians (Fleisch 1991). In brief, bisphosphonates inhibit bone resorption in cell and organ cultures, irrespective of whether bone resorption is stimulated or not. They also prevent experimentally induced bone resorption very effectively. The potency of different bisphosphonates to inhibit bone resorption varies from one for etidronate to approximately 10,000 for zoledronate. Potencies found in the rat model and in human beings are comparable. The P-C-P structure appears to be a necessary prerequisite for the activity. However, the intensity of the effect is dependent on the side chain (Shinoda et al. 1983). Furthermore, recent investigations have shown that stereoisomeres of the same chemical structure differ up to tenfold in their activity. This implies that some kind of receptor properties may exist in the mediation of at least a part of the bisphosphonate activity. Further research in this area is needed to clarify the question (Fleisch 1995). Having covered the bone surface, the bisphosphonates are buried in the skeleton under new layers of bone. Bisphosphonates may be liberated again by physicochemical mechanisms and when bone is resorbed. Their half-life in the body therefore

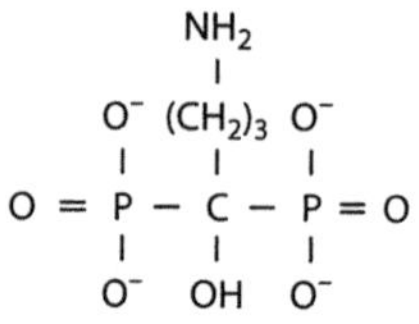

(4-Amino-1-hydroxybutylidene)-
bis-phosphonate

alendronate*

Gentili; Merck Sharp & Dohme)

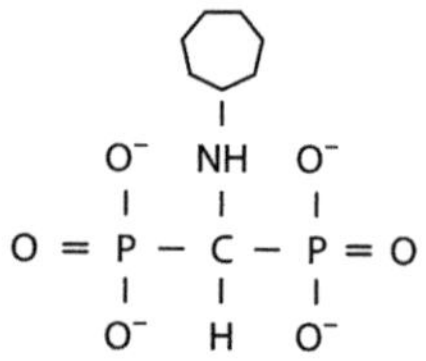

[(Cycloheptylamino)-
methylene]bis-phosphonate

cimadronate

Yamanouchi

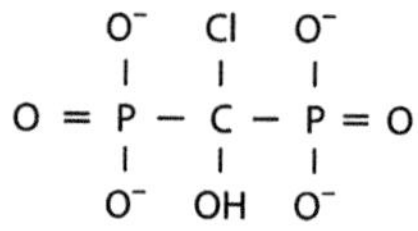

(Dichloromethylene)-
bis-phosphonate

clodronate*

*Astra; Boehringer Mannheim;
Gentili; Leiras; Rhône-Poulenc Rorer*

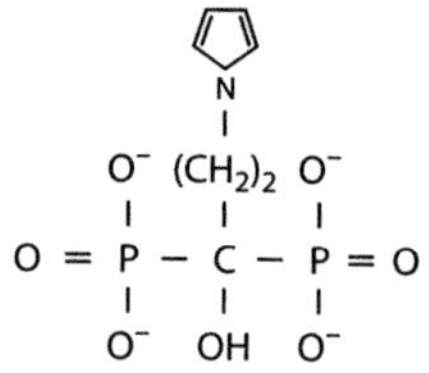

[1-Hydroxy-3-(1-pyrrolidinyl)-
propylidene]bis-phosphonate

EB-1053

Leo

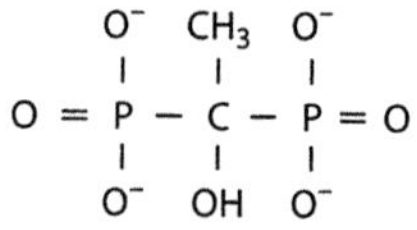

(1-hydroxyethylidene)-
bis-phosphonate

etidronate*

Gentili; Procter & Gamble

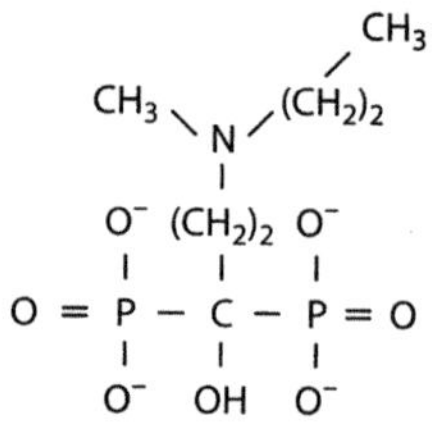

[1-Hydroxy-3-(methylpentylamino)
propylidene]bis-phosphonate

ibandronate*

Boehringer Mannheim

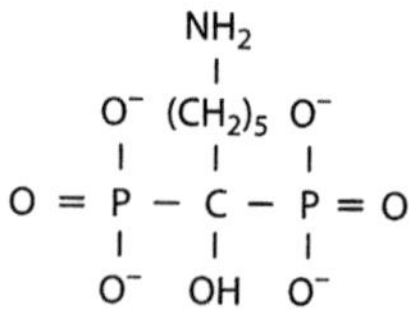

(6-Amino-1-hydroxyhexy-
lidene)bis-phosphonate

neridronate

Gentili

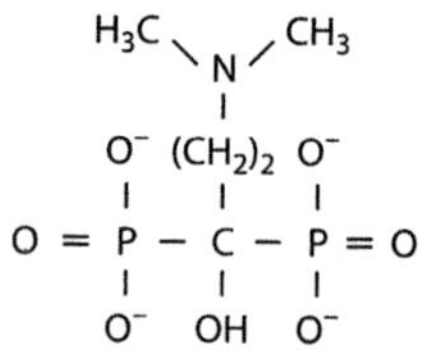

[3-(Dimethylamino)-1-hdroxy-
propylidene]bis-phosphonate

olpadronate

Gador

Fig. 1.

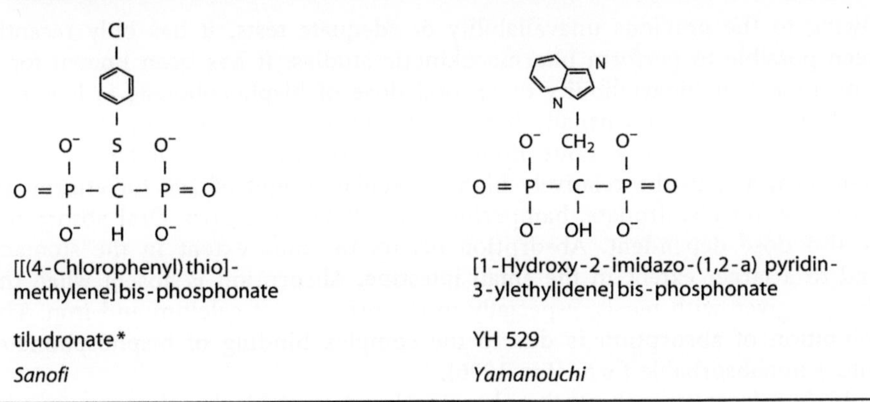

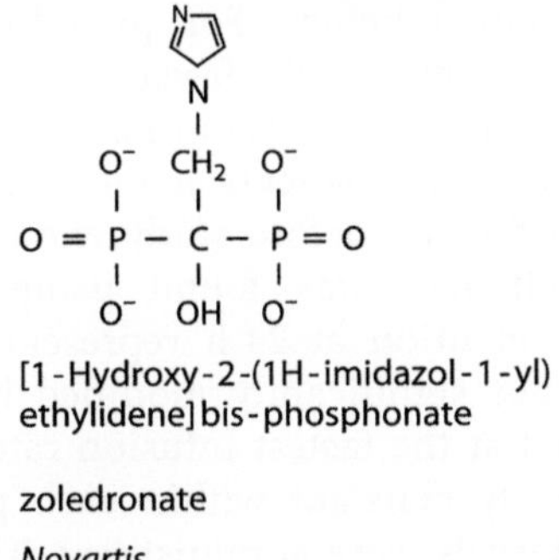

(3-Amino-1-hydroxypropy-
lidene)bis-phosphonate

pamidronate*

Novartis; Gador

[1-Hydroxy-2-(3-pyridinyl)-
ethylidene]bis-phosphonate

risedronate

Procter & Gamble

[[(4-Chlorophenyl)thio]-
methylene]bis-phosphonate

tiludronate*

Sanofi

[1-Hydroxy-2-imidazo-(1,2-a) pyridin-
3-ylethylidene]bis-phosphonate

YH 529

Yamanouchi

[1-Hydroxy-2-(1H-imidazol-1-yl)
ethylidene]bis-phosphonate

zoledronate

Novartis

Fig. 1. Chemical structures of bisphosphonates used in human beings. *Asterisks* indicate a product that is commercially available. (From H. Fleisch)

depends to a large extent on the rate of bone turnover. As the bisphosphonates decrease resorption and thus slower bone turnover, their half-life may be even longer than that of the untreated skeleton. Bone turnover is much slower in human beings than in mice or rats. Therefore, data obtained from animal models cannot be easily extrapolated to humans. It is possible that at least a proportion of administered bisphosphonate remains in the body for the life of an individual. This is also observed with other substances which are buried in bone such as tetracyclines, fluoride, strontium, and phosphate.

Pharmacokinetics

Owing to the previous unavailability of adequate tests, it has only recently been possible to perform pharmacokinetic studies. It has been known for a long time that bioavailibility of an oral dose of bisphosphonate is low, certainly below 10% and usually between 1 and 3%. This low rate is likely attributable to the very poor lipophility, preventing transcellular intestinal transport, and to the relatively high molecular weight of 206 for etidronate, up to 249 for alendronate, hampering paracellular transport. Oral absorption is also dose dependent. Absorption occurs to some extent in the stomach and to a larger extent in the small intestine. Absorption is absent when the drug is given with meals, especially in the presence of calcium and iron. The inhibition of absorption is due to the complex binding of bisphosphonates into a nonabsorbable form (Lin 1996).

Little information about the pharmacokinetics of bisphosphonates in man is available, as mentioned before. For pamidronate, the mean 24-h body retention values in patients with fewer than five bone metastases was $50.6\pm11.8\%$, and it reached $76.4\pm12\%$ in patients with more than 15 metastases. In a subgroup of seven patients a more accurate count was made by bone scintigraphy performed before study entry. In this group of patients a high correlation coefficient was found using linear regression analysis ($r=0.82$). The body retention at 24 h represented 60–70% of the administered dose and was not significantly modified by the infusion rate and, in particular, not reduced at the fastest infusion rate (1 mg/h) tested; 24-h body retention was practically constant within each patient when repeated infusions at 4–5 week intervals were administered. These results suggest that the bone compartment was not saturated after repeated infusions – as expected from animal models. Tolerance was excellent except for one patient who developed phlebitis at the infusion site. In particular, no renal toxicity was observed with one to four infusions. On the basis of this study, the 1-h infusion time was proposed as appropriate for the administration of 60 mg pamidronate to patients with metastatic bone disease and normal or slightly reduced renal function. More detailed results of these pharmacokinetic studies are reported elsewhere (Leyvraz et al. 1992).

Distribution

In human beings, of any given dose, about 20% of clodronate, 50% of etidronate, and 70% of alendronate or pamidronate are bound to the skeleton. A small proportion is bound to proteins, especially albumin. The remainder is rapidly excreted in the urine. The deposition is proportionally greater when large amounts of the compounds are given (Lin et al. 1994). However, large quantities should not be infused rapidly because this can cause the formation of aggregates and complexes which may cause renal failure. The half-life of circulating bisphosphonates is in the range of 0.5–2 h. Bone clearance is compatible with a complete extraction by the skeleton after the first passage. The areas of deposition are generally thought to be mostly those of active bone formation. This property is visualized in areas with high bone turnover by means of ^{99m}Tc-linked bisphosphonates. When bisphosphonates are given to human beings in clinical doses by repeated infusions there seems to be no saturation of the skeleton. However, after long-term continuous administration the accumulation in the skeleton reaches a plateau. The plateau effect is dose dependent. The reason for this discrepancy between the time required for maximal incorporation of the drug and that required for its maximal effect is unclear, but it may be due to the unequal distribution within the skeleton.

References

Fleisch H (1991) Bisphosphonates: pharmacology and use in the treatment of tumor induced hypercalcemia metastatic bone disease. Drugs 42:919–944

Fleisch H (1995) Relative activity of bisphosphonates. In: Fleisch H (ed) Bisphosphonates in bone disease: from the laboratory to the patient, 2nd edn. Parthenon, Lancs, pp 38–58

Leyvraz S, Hess U, Flesh G, Bauer J, Hauffe S, Ford JM, Burckhardt P (1992) Pharmacokinectics of pamidronate in patients with bone metastases. J Natl Cancer Inst 84:788–792

Lin JH (1996) Bisphosphonates: a review of their pharmacokinectic properties. Bone 18:75–85

Lin JH, Chen IW, de Luna FA (1994) On the absorption of alendronate in rats. J Pharm Sci 83:1741–1746

Shinoda H, Adamek G, Felix R, Fleisch H, Schenk R, Hagan P (1983) Structure activity relationships of various bisphosphonates. Calcif Tissue Int 35:87–99

Hypercalcemia of Malignancy

Magnitude of the Problem

The association of hypercalcemia and malignancy was first reported in 1924 (Zondek et al. 1924). The syndrome of humeral hypercalcemia of cancer was first described in 1941 (Case records of the Massachusetts General Hospital 1941). The authors reported a temporary correction of hypercalcemia and hypophosphatemia after radiation of bone metastases from a renal carcinoma and hypothesized that the tumor was secreting PTH or a peptide with similar action. This hypothesis was later supported by two studies that described a series of patients who had hypercalcemia in the absence of skeletal tumor involvement or whose hypercalcemia was corrected by eliminating the tumor (Plimpton and Gellhorn 1956; Connor et al. 1956). In 1966, the term pseudohyperparathyroidism was used to describe a series of 50 such patients and to propose a set of diagnostic criteria (Lafferty 1966), but only in 1988, following intensive investigation of humeral hypercalcemia of malignancy, and as a result of the clear biochemical characterization of the syndrome, was the peptide called "parathyroid hormone-like peptide" (PTH-rP) identified (Proadus et al. 1988).

The recognition of hypercalcemia has been facilitated by the introduction of routine analysis of the serum calcium levels in blood biochemistry examinations. The incidence of hypercalcemia of malignancy is estimated to be about 15 per 100,000 population per year. Among 207 consecutive patients with hypercalcemia, 72 with hypercalcemia of malignancy were detected. Although hypercalcemia of malignancy is less frequent than primary hyperparathyroidism among the general population, it is obviously more frequently detected in the hospital population, as patients with primary hyperparathyroidism are usually asymptomatic and, if recognized, are treated as outpatients, whereas patients with tumor-induced hypercalcemia are frequently symptomatic and are hospitalized due to poor general condition with far advanced malignant disease. Prior to the development of potent second-seneration bisphosphonates patients usually were also admitted for treatment with rehydration and plicamycin (Mundy et al. 1980; Mundy and Martin 1982).

The body defenses against hypercalcemia caused by bone destruction or large dietary calcium load include (a) a decrease in PTH secretion, but only up to a serum calcium concentration of 2.9 mmol/l; (b) calcitonin, which is very effective, but has no long-term efficacy; and (c) vitamin D_3, whose effects are slow and limited. Furthermore, the filtered load of calcium increases with glomerular filtration and a possible diuretic effect of hypercalcemia eventually leading to sodium and volume depletion, a transient effect which finally leads to decreased calcium excretion. Overall, the body's defenses against hypocalcemia and its consequences seem to be much better than those against hypercalcemia.

Pathogenesis

Although hypercalcemia can occur in virtually any tumor, some tumors cause hypercalcemia more frequently than others, most commonly breast cancer and myeloma, lung cancers and uroepithelial cancers, whereas adenocarcinomas of the gastrointestinal tract rarely cause hypercalcemia (Mundy and Martin 1982). For many years hypercalcemia of malignancy was considered to be the result of excessive release of skeletal calcium by bone metastases, while hypercalcemia in the small group of patients without bone lesions was attributed to systemic release of humeral hypercalcemic factors. This concept had to be revised on the basis of studies done in the 1980s. No significant correlation was found between extent of bone metastases and serum calcium values in cancer patients (Ralston et al. 1987). Biochemical evaluation revealed evidence of an underlying humeral etiology in the majority of hypercalcemic cancer patients (Stuart et al. 1980; Ralston et al. 1984). Furthermore, evaluation of patients with metastatic bone disease has shown that amounts of calcium released by metastases alone are insufficient to cause hypercalcemia unless normal homeostatic mechanisms for calcium excretion are also impaired (Ralston et al. 1984). This endocrine effect on renal calcium reabsorption indicates that in the majority of cases humoral factors are most important for hypercalcemia, irrespective of the presence or absence of bone metastases.

Mediators

In breast cancer hypercalcemia often develops in patients with very advanced disease and extensive bone involvement. In these patients local osteolysis may also be an important pathogenetic mechanism, combined with other factors such as sodium depletion (Hosking et al. 1981) and immobilization (Ralston et al. 1989a). Paracrine mediators of osteolysis have been described above. Procathepsin D secreted by human breast cancer cells seems also to contribute to osteoclast activation (Wo et al. 1989). However, in 50–60% of cases PTH-rP can be found in the serum (Isales et al. 1987; Percival et al. 1985).

In solid tumors other than breast cancer, PTH-rP is the principal cause of hypercalcemia. A few patients with solid tumors and hypercalcemia in the absence of bone metastases do not show biochemical evidence of PTH-rP excess. In these patients, prostaglandin-stimulating factors may be involved in the pathogenesis of hypercalcemia (Bringhurst et al. 1986). In such cases prostaglandin synthetase inhibitors may be successful in correcting hypercalcemia (Seyberth et al. 1975). In myeloma, hypercalcemia is associated with increased bone resorption due to the widespread osteolytic process and renal impairment, which is most probably due to effects of Bence-Jones protein on the kidney. The predominant osteolytic mediators have already been described. In malignant lymphoma various mechanisms contribute to hypercalcemia. Local release of paracrine factors, as mentioned above, and excessive production of vitamin D_3 have been described in patients with lymphoma, including those with Hodgkins' disease (Davies et al. 1985).

Treatment

Obviously, the best long-term results are obtained by treating the tumor itself with antineoplastic medications. However, such treatment can be offered to only a minority of hypercalcemic patients. Among these are patients who present with hypercalcemia as the first symptom of their disease. Patients with multiple myeloma, hypercalcemia, and impaired renal function constitute the majority within this minority of hypercalcemic patients. Less frequently seen are patients with the onset of metastatic disease following primary treatment for early breast cancer. Also breast cancer patients with extensive bone involvement who are receiving tamoxifen as first-line hormone therapy for advanced disease can develop hypercalcemia.

For the vast majority of patients, antihypercalcemic treatment begins with correction of the extracellular fluid deficit. Rehydration alone may normalize serum calcium in some patients with mild hypercalcemia. Transient reduction of serum calcium values by about 0.5 mmol/l can be achieved in patients with moderate hypercalcemia. However, in patients with rapidly progressive disease and severe hypercalcemia, serum calcium values may increase during the first 48 h, even with adequate intravenous fluid intake (Thürlimann 1994; Pechersdorfer et al. 1996; Boehringer Mannheim 1996: data on file).

Today, treatment with bisphosphonates is usually initiated concomitantly with rehydration in all hypercalcemic patients with adequate renal function (e.g., creatinine clearance should be <350 μmol/l for slow infusion of pamidronate). However, in patients with further impairment of kidney function pamidronate has to be administered with caution and infusion time has to be prolonged. In patients with life-threatening hypercalcemia, antihypercalcemic treatment that acts on renal calcium excretion should be started immediately after the diagnosis has been made and administration of adequate fluid must be initiated. Calcitonin has proven to be very useful in this situation, lowering serum calcium within 2 h of starting therapy (Wisneski et al. 1978). Although tachyphylaxis to this treatment is well known, the drug can usually control hypercalcemia adequately and thus buy time for other more potent osteoclast inhibitors such as bisphosphonates. Intravenous phosphate should not be used except when calcitonin is ineffective. Rapid infusion must be avoided, especially in patients with preexisting hyperphosphatemia and renal impairment. It lowers serum calcium within minutes due to formation of insoluble calcium phosphate complexes. As previously described, these complexes can lead to tissue calcification and death due to acute renal failure or hypotension (Breuer and LeBauer 1967).

Rehydration and Supportive Care

Rehydration, supportive care, and plicamycin have constituted the standard treatment for tumor-associated hypercalcemia for more than 20 years in oncology departments (Senn and Peyer 1978; Perlia et al. 1970). Glucocorticoids were often used but had not proven to be effective except in hypercalcemia associated with hematological malignancies (Binstock and Mundy 1980; Thalassinos and Joplin 1970; Mundy et al. 1970; Percival et al. 1984).

Forced diuresis in conjunction with high doses of furosemide has also been used (Suki et al. 1970). Although hydration and administration of furosemide in much smaller doses than recommended in the previously mentioned reference have been a very fashionable therapy for the treatment of hypercalcemia of malignancy in the USA (Mundy 1989), the only evidence of usefulness of this therapy came from the aforementioned study, in which 16 patients with hypercalcemia were treated with 100 mg furosemide every 2 h. A considerable but transient fall in serum calcium was obtained. All of the patients received fluid in addition to furosemide, and it was impossible to distinguish the effects of fluid intake from those of furosemide. Furthermore, in patients who are not yet fully rehydrated, furosemide may be likely to worsen the hypercalcemia due to further depletion of extracellular fluid volume. This effect will cause even more calcium reabsorption in patients who already have increased calcium reabsorption from the proximal convoluted tubule. On the other hand, overhydration of patients who require fluid therapy is often observed in hospitals and can lead to cardiac failure and pulmonary edema, especially in the elderly (Senn and Peyer 1987).

Plicamycin (Mithramycin)

Plicamycin was developed from *Streptomyces plicatus*, a fungus-like bacterium of the family Streptomycetaceae, order Actinomycetales. Its chemical structure and mechanism of action are similar to those of actinomycin D. It acts as an RNA synthesis inhibitor (Au Yarbro et al. 1966). Plicamycin was developed as a cytotoxic drug during the 1960s and was successfully used in the treatment of disseminated testicular cancer (Kofman et al. 1964; Brown and Kennedy 1965). Many testicular cancer patients treated with plicamycin suffered also from a profound drop in serum calcium. Because of this incidental finding, plicamycin was used in many oncology centers as an empiric antihypercalcemic drug, and it remained the treatment of choice for over two decades. No general agreement on how to best use plicamycin had been reached, but most clinicians gave an initial infusion of about 20 µg/kg body wt. and then waited to see whether there was a fall in calcium. If the effect was insufficient or if calcium increased again, the treatment could be repeated. Plicamycin's maximal effect together with rehydration occurred about 3–4 days after the infusion, but some patients did not achieve normal calcium, and relapse within a few days was frequent (Mundy et al. 1983). Moreover, plicamycin was also associated with considerable toxicity. It caused nausea and vomiting and liver damage, leading to increased hepatocellular enzymes. Its nephrotoxicity, a serious disadvantage to its use in this patient population in which many individuals already have impaired renal function, was certainly disadvantageous. Plicamycin can cause bone marrow toxicity and severe thrombocytopenia. Moreover, it may further impair thrombocyte function and the coagulation and fibrinolytic process, thus increasing further the risk of bleeding, especially when administered repeatedly, as its toxic effects may accumulate (Gasser et al. 1974; Monto et al. 1969; Ahr et al. 1987; Ashby and Lazarchick 1986). Serious life-threatening side effects and death have been reported after a single infusion of plicamycin. It should be used only in patients with normal or near-normal renal function and there should be close monitoring of liver function tests, daily blood counts, and renal function tests. In our experience and that of many others, when plicamycin is completely ineffective, so too are most other hypercalcemic drugs (Mundy 1990; Thürlimann, own observations).

Dialysis

Both peritoneal dialysis (Miach et al. 1975) and hemodialysis (Kaiser et al. 1989; Strauch and Ball 1976; Cardella et al. 1979; Leow and Wagner 1973) have also been used for more than 20 years. Obviously, dialysis is not an effective long-term form of treatment for hypercalcemia, because increased bone resorption is not counteracted. Severe complications during hemodialysis were also reported (Kaiser et al. 1989). Dialysis is indicated mainly when other forms of treatment are contraindicated or ineffective and when the patient has a reversible form of renal failure.

Bisphosphonates

Bisphosphonates are the most effective drugs and the treatment of choice for tumor-induced hypercalcemia. In 1972, etidronate and clodronate were reported to have similar calcium-lowering effects (Jung 1972). Etidronate is given by slow intravenous infusion, and previous high-dose regimens are no longer used because of the risk of acute renal failure (Bounamaux et al. 1983). The recommended dose is 7.5 mg/kg body wt. per day for 3 consecutive days (Hasling et al. 1987). Continuation of the treatment for up to 5 days does not seem to improve the results (Kanis et al. 1987). Although total serum calcium values normalize in 75–90% of the patients, the albumin corrected values, which more accurately reflect the physiologically important ionized calcium, are normalized in only about 25–30% of cases (Kanis et al. 1987; Ralston et al. 1989b). The effect of etidronate lasts about 10–12 days (Ralston et al. 1989b; Ringerberg and Ritch 1987). Successful maintenance therapy has been reported by some investigators (Ringerberg and Ritch 1987), but others have been disappointed (Ralston et al. 1989b).

Clodronate is a slightly more potent inhibitor of bone resorption than etidronate in vitro. Various dose regimens of clodronate have been used. Current evidence suggests that there is little clinically relevant difference between the regimens. About 40% of patients became normocalcemic with a single dose of 600 mg clodronate (Ralston et al. 1989; Adami et al. 1987). The oral formulation of clodronate is also effective in some cases (Adami et al. 1987; Chapuy et al. 1980).

Various regimens of pamidronate have been examined, using daily doses of 15 mg once up to a total of 150 mg and single infusions of between 5 and 90 mg (Sleeboom et al. 1983; Ralston et al. 1985, 1990; Thiébaud et al. 1986 a; Coleman and Rubens 1987; Morton et al. 1988; Nussbaum et al. 1989). Most clinicians use pamidronate according to the calcium level at the beginning of antihypercalcemic treatment. Many patients with mild hypercalcemia respond adequately to doses of 30 mg. Serum calcium will normalize in about 80–90% of patients with doses of 60 mg (Thürlimann et al. 1992). Only in patients with severe hypercalemia (>4 mmol/l) or recurrent hypercalcemia may 90 mg of pamidronate be needed for adequate response. Oral formulations of pamidronate have also been used successfully (Thiébaud et al. 1986 b). However, the treatment is inconvenient, due to the fact that a well-tolerated oral formulation has not been developed. Pamidronate came from experimental, and later from clinical, endocrinologists to medical oncologists and had to establish its superiority to plicamycin, an antihypercalcemic treatment frequently used in most cancer centers during the 1970s and 1980s.

Plicamycin and Pamidronate in Symptomatic Tumor-related Hypercalcemia: A Prospective, Randomized Crossover Trial Conducted at the Department of Internal Medicine C, Kantonsspital, St. Gallen, and at the Department of Internal Medicine, CHUV, Lausanne, Switzerland[1]

In 1986 we knew from studies performed at the CHUV by Thiébaud and Burckardt and their co-workers that a single infusion of pamidronate 60 mg given over 24 h had proven to be simple, safe, and effective in the treatment of tumor-related hypercalcemia (Thiébaud et al. 1986 a). These results set the basis for comparing pamidronate and plicamycin, which had been the standard treatment for tumor-associated hypercalcemia for more than 20 years at our institution and at most other oncology units throughout the world. One year earlier, a comparison between pamidronate, mitramycin, and corticosteroids/calcitonin in the treatment of cancer-associated hypercalcemia had been published, but it remains unclear how mitramycin was administered in this study. From the report, it seems that there were no prospective determined doses specified when the treatment was started. The article reported rather a comparative trial of three different empirical strategies (Ralston et al. 1985). However, the results were encouraging enough for us to undertake a randomized study in our institution, testing prospectively specified doses of both pamidronate and plicamycin.

[1] B. Thürlimann, R. Waldburger, H.J. Senn, D. Thiébaud (1992) *Annals of Oncology* 3: 619–623; reproduced here, slightly modified, with kind permission from Kluwer Academic Publishers.

Patients and Methods

Eligibility

Criteria for inclusion of a patient in the study were histologically or cytologically proven malignancy and a first occurrence of symptomatic hypercalcemia, with a serum calcium level $\geqslant 2.8$ mmol/l corrected for total serum protein (upper limit in our institution is 2.5 mmol/l). Patients considered terminally ill and those with a serum creatinine level above 350 μmol/l were not eligible. Informed consent was obtained from all participating patients.

Study Design

Patients were enrolled in this study between May 1, 1987, and July 31, 1989. All study patients were hospitalized. Routine evaluation consisted of a complete blood cell count and assessment of serum electrolytes, including calcium, total protein, creatinine, blood urea nitrogen, bilirubin, AST, ALT, GGT, and alkaline phosphatase. Chest X-ray and electrocardiograms (ECGs) were also performed. Antihypercalcemic drug treatment was started immediately after the diagnosis of hypercalcemia had been confirmed, with no delay for rehydration. Random treatment assignment was based upon prepared envelopes. Entry into the two arms of the study was balanced within the two participating centers of the Department of Internal Medicine C, Division of Oncology, Kantonsspital St. Gallen (KSSG) and the Department of Internal Medicine, University Hospital Lausanne (CHUV).

In addition to the assigned calcium-lowering agent, each patient received more than 2000 ml 0.9% NaCl per day, continuing until serum calcium levels returned to normal. Pamidronate (APD) was supplied by Ciba Geigy, Basel, Switzerland, as disodium 3-amino-1-hydroxypropylidene-bisphosphonate pentahydrate (Aredia®) and was given in 1000 ml 0.9% NaCl by continuous intravenous infusion over 24 h at a dose of 60 mg, irrespective of body wt. and calcemia value. Plicamycin was administered intravenously for 30 min at a dose of 25 μg/kg body wt.

Serum calcium levels were ascertained daily during the first 7 days of the study. However, if normocalcemia was achieved within 1 week, determinations were permitted every second day. Thereafter, serum calcium levels were determined weekly until day 90 or death.

Resistance was defined as failure to lower the serum calcium level to 2.6 mmol/l or less after 6 days of treatment. Recurrence was defined as a further episode of hypercalcemia (serum calcium ≥ 2.8 mmol/l) within the 90-day observation period following normalization of the serum calcium level after the first treatment. Permanent response was defined as normalization of the serum calcium level without recurrence of hypercalcemia within the observation period, or until death from some other cause.

No systemic anticancer therapy was given during the first 6 days of the therapy for hypercalcemia unless the attending physician was convinced of its necessity before the serum calcium level and/or the creatinine level had normalized. Emergency chemotherapy prior to day 7 was administered to a total of eight patients (four patients in each of the two arms). In patients with resistant or recurrent hypercalcemia in whom a second antihypercalcemic treatment was indicated, the alternative drug was administered.

Statistical Considerations

The objective of the study was to evaluate the effectiveness and tolerability of the two treatments. Qualitative parameters were analyzed using the Student's t-test to compare mean values. The F-test compared standard deviations. Kendall's coefficient of concordance W-test was used additionally for all parameters with a large standard deviation, e.g., white cell count, which ranged from $2.2 \times 10^9/l$ to $32.0 \times 10^9/l$. In performing such an analysis, we replaced the data obtained with rank numbers and investigated whether the chronological course of these rank numbers showed a trend. If a trend was found, homogeneity of these trends and differences between treatment groups was further investigated. The likelihood-χ^2 test was used for statistical analysis of the qualitative parameters.

Results

A total of 48 patients with cancer and a first occurrence of symptomatic hypercalcemia were entered in the randomized trial. One patient had insufficient documentation and was therefore not evaluable. Three patients had concomitant primary hyperparathyroidism (later confirmed intraoperatively in two cases and at autopsy in one case), but since they met all study entry criteria, they were regarded as evaluable and included in the intention-to-treat analysis.

The mean age of the patients was 62 years (range 27–85 years), and the mean pretreatment total protein-corrected serum calcium level was 3.38 mmol/l; 58% of the patients had abnormal serum creatinine levels. Statistical analysis of the pretreatment characteristics (histology, age, serum calcium, serum creatinine, presence of bone metastases) showed no statistically significant differences between the two groups. Mean oral and intravenous fluid intake in the first 72 h after initiation of treatment was 9.26 l ($\pm$2.42 l) in the plicamycin group and 9.74 l ($\pm$2.4 l) in the pamidronate group ($p = 0.19$). Details are shown in Table 1.

Effectiveness

Both agents lowered serum calcium levels significantly. Between day 1 and day 7, ten of 22 evaluable patients (45%) who were randomized to the plicamycin group and 22 of 25 evaluable patients (88%) in the pamidronate group achieved normocalcemia ($p<0.01$). Analysis on day 7 revealed that ten of 21 evaluable patients (48%) in the plicamycin group and 19 of 22 (86%) in the pamidronate group had normal serum calcium levels ($p<0.01$).

If patients who received chemotherapy before day 7 are excluded from analysis, six of 18 patients (33%) in the plicamycin group and 19 of 21 patients (90%) in the pamidronate group achieved normocalcemia between day

Table 1. Patient characteristics[a]

	All patients ($n = 48$)	Plicamycin group ($n = 23$)	Pamidronate group ($n = 25$)
Mean age (years)	62.0	62.9	61.2
Sex, n (%)			
Male	20 (42)	10 (43)	10 (40)
Female	28 (58)	13 (57)	15 (60)
Tumor site/type, n (%)			
Breast	13 (27)	5 (22)	8 (32)
Lung	11 (23)	6 (26)	5 (20)
Myeloma	8 (17)	3 (13)	5 (20)
Unknown primary	5 (10)	2 (9)	3 (12)
Genitourinary	5 (10)	1 (4)	4 (16)
Gastrointestinal	4 (8)	4 (17)	0
Sarcoma	1 (2)	1 (4)	0
Prostate	1 (2)	1 (4)	0
Mean corrected serum calcium before treatment (mmol/l, ±SE)	3.38 (±0.41)	3.42 (±0.43)	3.35 (±0.3)
Mean serum creatinine before treatment (μmol/l, ±SE)	153 (±10.1)	163 (±10.6)	145 (±7.0)
Abnormal serum creatinine (>120 μmol/l) before treatment, n (%)	28 (58)	14 (61)	14 (56)
Mean SAKK-ECOG performance status at start of treatment	2.9	2.8	2.9
Bone metastases			
Present, n (%)	37 (77)	15 (65)	22 (88)
Absent, n (%)	11 (23)	8 (35)	3 (12)

[a] There was no significant difference between the treatment groups in any selection parameter.

1 and day 7. Eight of 21 patients (38%) in the plicamycin group and 14 of 22 pamidronate-treated patients (64%) remained normocalcemic during the study period of 90 days or until death from some other cause ($p<0.05$). Mean serum calcium reduction in the first 7 days after treatment was significantly more pronounced in the pamidronate-treated group. On day 7, the mean reduction was 0.67 ± 0.57 mmol/l in the plicamycin group and 1.09 ± 0.37 mmol/l in the pamidronate group ($p<0.01$). The difference in reduction of serum calcium became significant ($p<0.01$) after 4 days of treatment. The course of calcemia over time can be seen in Fig. 2. Patients in the pamidronate group experienced a significant decrease in serum creatinine levels within 1 week after treatment ($p<0.05$), whereas mean serum creatinine levels did not change in those receiving plicamycin (Fig. 3). Twelve patients in each group had elevated serum creatinine levels before treatment. In three of the latter patients (25%) treated with plicamycin and in seven of those (58%) treated with pamidronate, serum creatinine levels normalized within 1 week. This difference did not reach statistical significance.

In one cancer patient with primary hyperparathyroidism, the serum calcium level normalized within 3 days following infusion of plicamycin (cal-

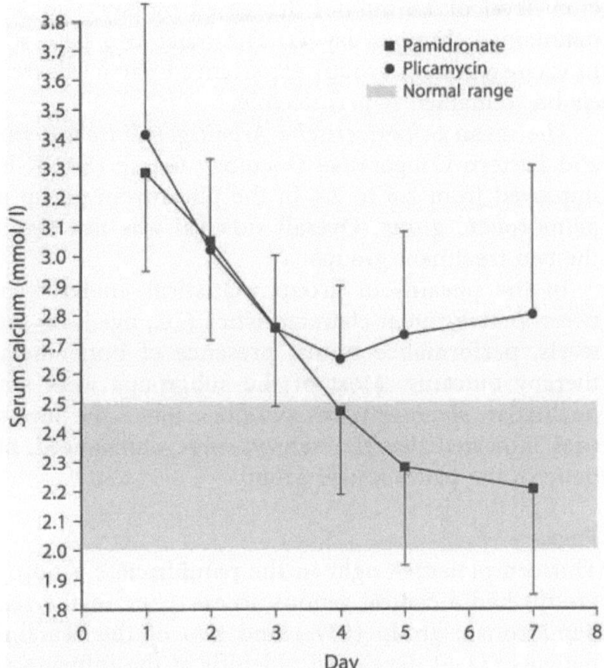

Fig. 2. Mean corrected serum calcium levels in patients with hypercalcemia of malignancy following treatment with plicamycin or pamidronate. Mean serum calcium reduction was significantly greater in pamidronate-treated patients 4 days after treatment ($p<0.01$)

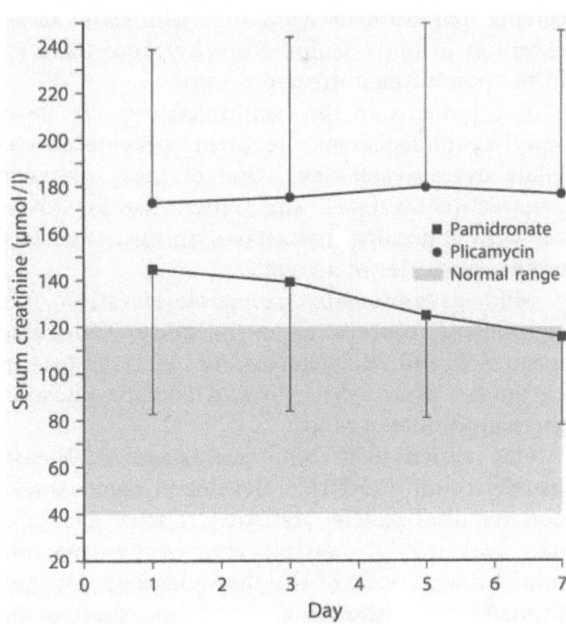

Fig. 3. Mean serum creatinine levels following treatment with plicamycin or pamidronate. Patients in the pamidronate group showed a significant decrease in mean serum creatinine within 1 week of treatment ($p<0.05$)

cium level of 3.4 mmol/l decreased by day 3 to 2.4 mmol/l, a level that was maintained through day 7). The other two patients with this condition (one in each treatment group) experienced partial decreases in serum calcium levels but remained hypercalcemic.

The mean *Schweizerische Arbeitsgemeinschaft für Klinische Krebsforschung* and Eastern Cooperative Oncology Group (SAKK-ECOG) performance status improved from 2.8 to 2.4 in the plicamycin group and from 2.9 to 2.4 in the pamidronate group. Overall survival was not significantly different between the two treatment groups.

In the plicamycin group, statistical analysis showed no correlation between pretreatment characteristics (i.e., age, sex, serum calcium or creatinine levels, performance status, presence of bone metastases, or histology) and therapy outcome. Most of the subgroups were small, and therefore only a qualitative statement was possible. Since the low number of treatment failures indicated that the subsets were unbalanced, statistical analysis was not done in the pamidronate group.

Toxicity

Thirteen patients (eight in the pamidronate group and five in the plicamycin group) had a central venous access. Nine of the remaining 17 patients in the pamidronate group (53%) and two of the remaining 18 plicamycin-treated patients (11%) developed phlebitis at the infusion site within 48 h after initiation of therapy ($p<0.05$). Vomiting occurred in eight of 22 evaluable patients (36%) in the plicamycin group but in none of 25 evaluable patients receiving pamidronate ($p<0.01$). Clinically asymptomatic hypocalcemia and elevation of body temperature by more than 1°C were observed more often in the pamidronate-treated group.

Two patients in the pamidronate group developed hypocalcemia and severe hypophosphatemia requiring parenteral replacement of calcium or phosphate over several days. One of these patients developed fatal necrotizing pancreatitis on day 4. This patient had far advanced non-small cell lung cancer with abdominal metastases and was known to regularly consume considerable quantities of alcohol.

Mild, asymptomatic, reversible elevation of liver function tests was seen significantly more often in the plicamycin-treated group ($p<0.01$) On day 3, mean AST and ALT values were twice the pretreatment levels in the plicamycin group. Mean AST, ALT and alkaline phosphatase remained unchanged in the pamidronate group.

One patient with bone metastases of breast cancer and a pretreatment platelet count of 54×10^9/l developed severe thrombocytopenia (nadir, 5×10^9/l) and required platelet transfusion after plicamycin infusion. Another patient had fatal arterial bleeding from a duodenal ulcer following plicamycin administration. None of the three patients with thrombocytopenia in the pamidronate group showed a significant drop in platelet count after treatment. For details of toxicity see Table 2.

Table 2. Side effects of plicamycin and pamidronate

	Patients (%)	Plicamycin (%)	Pamidronate (%)	p-value
Vomiting	$n=47$	$n=22$	$n=25$	
Mild	3 (7)	3 (14)	0	
Moderate	4 (8)	4 (18)	0	<0.01
Severe	1 (2)	1 (5)	0	
Absent	39 (83)	14 (63)	25 (100)	<0.01
Phlebitis at infusion site	$n=35$	$n=18$	$n=17$	<0.05
Present	11 (31)	2 (11)	9 (53)	
Absent	24 (69)	16 (89)	8 (47)	
Body temperature increase $\geq 1^\circ$C within 36 h of treatment	$n=47$	$n=11$	$n=25$	
Present	12 (26)	2 (9)	10 (40)	<0.01
Absent	35 (74)	20 (91)	15 (60)	<0.05
Hypocalcemia (calcium ≤ 2.0 mmol/l)	$n=47$	$n=22$	$n=25$	
Yes	9 (19)	1 (5)	8 (32)	<0.01
Mild (Ca ≤ 1.8)	8	1	7	
Moderate (Ca ≤ 1.5)	0	0	0	
Severe (Ca ≤ 1.4)	1	0	1	
No	38 (81)	21 (95)	17 (68)	

Crossover Treatment

Twenty patients showed resistance or recurrence of hypercalcemia after the first treatment. Twelve of these patients (ten plicamycin failures, two pamidronate failures) were treated with the alternative drug. As second-line therapy, pamidronate corrected the elevated serum calcium level in seven of the ten plicamycin failures, and plicamycin normalized the level in one of the two pamidronate failures. Asymptomatic elevation of body temperature by more than 1°C (in two of ten patients), asymptomatic hypocalcemia (in three of ten patients), and hypophosphatemia (in five of ten patients) were seen in pamidronate-treated patients only. Phlebitis developed in two of eight patients following administration of pamidronate and in one of two patients who received plicamycin as second-line therapy. Statistical analysis was not carried out because of the unbalanced groups and the small number of patients treated with pamidronate.

Discussion

In this study, a single intravenous 60-mg dose of pamidronate produced normalization of serum calcium levels in 22 of 25 (88%) hypercalcemic cancer patients. This high response rate is comparable to the results achieved with 60 mg of pamidronate in previously published phase-II studies (Cantwell and Harris 1986; Thiébaud et al. 1986a, 1988; Morton et al. 1988). In the present comparative study, plicamycin was significantly less effective than pamidronate, producing normalization of serum calcium in only ten of 22 patients (45%) ($p<0.01$). This comparative result is similar to that reported in a study in which plicamycin was administered by single or repeated injection (Ralston et al. 1985).

Similar results were later reported in a confirmatory Norwegian study: significantly more patients randomized to pamidronate achieved normocalcemia as compared with patients randomized to plicamycin. Mean serum calcium values on day 6 of treatment were 2.48 mmol/l versus 2.92 mmol/l ($p<0.05$) (Anderson and Ostenstad 1991).

The favorable results in our initial comparison of pamidronate and plicamycin were confirmed in the crossover phase of the study, in which pamidronate corrected the serum calcium elevation in seven of ten plicamycin failures. In addition to its superiority to plicamycin in the present study, pamidronate was reported to be superior to etidronate (7.5 mg/kg per day ×3) and clodronate (600 mg i.v.) in previously published reports (Ritch et al. 1992; Ralston et al. 1989b).

Pamidronate was well tolerated in the present comparative study. It did not cause emesis or abnormalities of bone marrow, liver, or kidney function. In our experience, pamidronate can be given safely and effectively in this patient population with creatinine levels as high as 350 µmol/l. The major subjective side effect of pamidronate was phlebitis at the infusion site in nine of 17 evaluable patients. The use of peripheral venous access catheters may have contributed to the development of phlebitis. In contrast, plicamycin therapy produced vomiting in eight of 22 evaluable patients (36%), and was associated with severe hematological and/or bleeding complications in two patients.

The 24-h infusion period for pamidronate administration was used in the present study because the vast majority of patients had symptomatic hypercalcemia and were hospitalized for rehydration. They had no urgent need for rapid infusion of pamidronate. Furthermore, no safety data allowing faster infusion of pamidronate were available at that point in time. Results from this study were not easily adapted to an outpatient setting. Studies performed later, at our institution and others, showed that 60 mg pamidronate can be administered intravenously over 2 h with acceptable tolerance in patients with malignant osteolytic bone disease (Hess et al. 1991). However, these patients usually have adequate renal function and are not volume depleted, in contrast to patients with tumor-induced hypercalcemia, as shown in our above-mentioned comparative study.

Other Bisphosphonates

Meanwhile, other second- and third-generation bisphosphonates have been tested and compared with other bisphosphonates in tumor-induced hypercalcemia. Aminobutane bisphosphonate, i.e., alendronate, has been investigated in dose-finding studies and compared with clodronate (Adami et al. 1987; Nussbaum et al. 1993; Rizzoli et al. 1992). YM175 was developed and tested in Japan (Fukumoto et al. 1994). Aminohexane bisphosphonate, i.e., Nenidronate, has also been examined in tumor-induced hypercalcemia (O'Rourke et al. 1994).

However, methylpentylaminopropylidene bisphosphonate, i.e., ibandronate (BM 21.0955), is clearly the third-generation bisphosphonate which is most developed and already registered in several countries for the treatment of tumor-induced hypercalcemia (Wüster et al. 1993). Our institution also contributed significantly to the development of ibandronate from the very beginning and participated actively in the pivotal multicenter trials, which included almost 300 patients. A dose-dependent response, defined as normalization of albumin-corrected serum calcium, was found in the first study. Doses of 2 mg were necessary to achieve a response rate comparable to that achieved with adequate doses of pamidronate or clodronate (Pechersdorfer et al. 1996).

In the consecutive study doses of 2, 4, and 6 mg were compared. The 2-mg dose was significantly less effective than the 4-mg and 6-mg doses. Normocalcemia was achieved in 76% and 78% with doses of 4 mg and 6 mg, respectively (Ralston 1996). Logistic regression analysis was performed in order to define parameters at baseline which were predictive for response. It was concluded that in patients with breast cancer and hematological malignancies with serum calcium ≤ 3.0 mmol/l, a dose of 2 mg is sufficient to achieve normocalcemia, while 4 mg is required for an optimal response with calcium values up to 3.5 mmol/l and 6 mg for calcium values above 3.5 mmol/l. Conversely, in patients with humoral hypercalcemia in other solid tumors, 6 mg is required for for serum calcium values >3 mmol/l (Ralston et al. 1997).

Zoledronate is the most potent bisphosphonate now in clinical development, and early results in hypercalcemia are promising (Lipton 1996). Later, the same group reported that the osteoclastic bone resorption as indicated by the biochemical markers PYD, DPD and NXT was significantly more inhibited by zoledronate 0.8 mg as compared to pamidronate 90 mg (Lipton 1998)

The last two bisphosphonates mentioned, i.e., ibandronate and zoldronate, can also be given as intravenous injection. The lack of toxicity of these newer compounds when administered as rapid infusion or injection gives them a considerable advantage with regard to practicability in the treatment of hypercalcemia. While this seems to be very important in the treatment and prevention of malignant osteolytic bone disease and osteoporosis, improvement of treatment by rapid administration of antihypercalcemic drugs is of limited value because the vast majority of patients with clinically relevant hypercalcemia of malignancy are hospitalized for other reasons, as mentioned above.

Gallium Nitrate

Gallium nitrate is an anticancer drug which causes hypocalcemia and increased urinary calcium excretion (Krakoff et al. 1979; Warrell et al. 1983). Only more recently was it found that the calcium-lowering effect of calcium nitrate meant decreased bone resorption (Warrell et al. 1984). Gallium nitrate was shown to be effective as a continuous intravenous infusion of 200 mg/m^2 daily for 5–7 days (Warrell et al. 1984) in later dose-finding studies. The superiority of 200 mg/m^2 was proved with regard to a prolonged effect on maintaining normocalcemia (Warrell et al. 1986). Later, several randomized double-blind studies revealed that, in doses of 200 mg/m^2 per day, gallium nitrate was more effective with regard to numbers of patients reaching normocalcemia and duration of normocalcemia as compared with calcitonin given intravenously in doses of 8 units/kg body wt. every 6 h for 5 days (Warrell et al. 1987). In another study, gallium nitrate was also more effective than etidronate in achieving a more prolonged drop in serum calcium levels. Gallium nitrate has never been investigated as widely as the bisphosphonates, especially in patients with impaired renal function. The most significant drawback is the requirement for a continuous infusion over several days. More convenient forms of drug administration such as subcutaneous injection are under investigation and may be found to be effective and useful.

Cisplatin

Cisplatin has also been used effectively in animal models of human hypercalcemia of malignancy (Kukla et al. 1984). It was shown to normalize serum calcium in a dose of 100 mg/m^2 in nine patients with malignant hypercalcemia for a rather long average duration of 38 days. No detectable reduction in tumor size was observed. However, cisplatin is not used in this indication because of its side effects such as nausea and vomiting and the potential nephrotoxic effect, especially in patients with impaired renal function (Kuckla et al. 1984; Lad et al. 1987).

References

Adami S, Wolzicci GP, Rizzo A, et al (1987) The use of dichloromethylene bisphosphonate and aminobutane bisphosphonates in hypercalcemia of malignancy. Bone Miner 2:395–404

Ahr DJ, Scialla SJ, Kiemball DB (1987) Acquired platelet dysfunction following mithramycin therapy. Cancer 41:448–454

Anderson OK, Ostenstad B (1991) Hypercalcemia of malignancy: mithramycin versus disodium pamidronate (APD), a randomised comparative trial. Eur J Cancer [Suppl] 2:abstract 1765

Ashby MA, Lazarchick J (1986) Acquired dysfibrinogenemia secondary to mithramycin therapy. Am J Med Sci 292:53–55

Au Yarbro JW, Kennedy BJ, Barnum CP (1966) Mithramycin inhibition of ribonucleic acid synthesis. Cancer Res 26:36–39

Binstock ML, Mundy GR (1980) Effect of calcitonin and glucocorticoids in combination in malignant hypercalcemia. Ann Intern Med 93:269–272

Bounamaux H, Schifferli I, Montany JB, Jung A, Chatelanat F (1983) Renal failure associated with intravenous bisphosphonates. Lancet 1:471

Breuer RI, LeBauer J (1967) Caution in the use of phosphates in the treatment of severe hypercalcemia. J Clin Endocrinol 27:695–698

Bringhurst FR, Bierer BE, Godeau F, Neyhard N, Varner V, Segre GV (1986) Tumoral hypercalcemia of malignancy: release of prostaglandin stimulating bone resorbing factor in vitro by human transitional carcinoma cells. J Clin Invest 77:456–464

Brown JH, Kennedy BJ (1965) Mithramycin in the treatment of disseminated testicular neoplasms. N Engl J Med 272:1011–1018

Cantwell B, Harris AL (1986) Single high dose aminohydroxy-propylidene diphosphonate infusions to treat cancer-associated hypercalcemia. Lancet 1:165–166

Cardella CJ, Birkin BL, Roscoe M, Rapaport A (1979) Role of dialysis in the treatment of severe hypercalcemia: report of two cases successfully treated with hemodialysis and review of the literature. Clin Nephrol 6:285–290

Case records of the Massachusetts General Hospital (1941) Case 27461. N Engl J Med 225:789–791

Chapuy MC, Meunier PJ, Alexandre C (1980) Effects of the disodium dichlormethylene bisphosphate on hypercalcemia produced by metastases. J Clin Invest 65:1243–1247

Coleman RE, Rubens RD (1987) (3-amino-1-hydroxypropylidene)-1,1-bisphosphonate (APD) for hypercalcemia of breast cancer. Br J Cancer 56:465–496

Connor TB, Thomas WC, Howard JF (1956) The etiology of hypercalcemia associated with lung carcinoma. J Clin Invest 35:697–698 (abstract)

Davies M, Hayes ME, Marwer EB, Lumb GA (1985) Abnormal vitamin D metabolism in Hodgkins' lymphoma. Lancet 2:1186–1188

Fukumoto S, Matsumoto T, Takebe K, Onaya T, Eto S, Nawata H, Ogata E (1994) Treatment of malignancy-associated hypercalcemia with YM175, a new bisphosphonate: elevated threshold for parathyroid hormone secretion in hypercalcemic patients. J Clin Endocrinol Metab 79:165–170

Gasser AB, Flury R, Senn HJ (1974) Therapie des Hyperkalzämie-Syndromes mit Mithramycin. Schweiz Med Wochenschr 104:1792

Hasling C, Charles P, Moseclide L (1987) Etidronate disodium in the management of malignancy-associated hypercalcemia. Am J Med 82:51–54

Hess U, Senn HJ, Ford J, et al (1991) Influence of infusion rate on pharmacokinetics of intravenous pamidronate (APD) in patients with bone metastases. In: Bijvoet O (ed) Proceedings of the international symposium on osteoclast inhibition in the management of malignancy-related bone disorders. Hamburg, Germany, 1991

Hosking DJ, Cowley A, Bucknall CA (1981) Rehydration in the treatment of severe hypercalcemia. Q J Med 200:473–481

Isales C, Carcangui ML, Stuart AF (1987) Hypercalcemia in breast cancer: re-evaluation. Am J Med 82:1143–1174

Jung A (1972) Comparison of two parenteral bisphosphates in hypercalcemia of malignancy. Ann Intern Med 29:923–930

Kaiser W, Biesenbach G, Kramer R, Zazkornik J (1989) Calcium-freie Hämodialyse-Stellenwert in der Therapie der hyperkalzämischen Krise. Klin Wochenschr 67:86–91

Kanis JA, Urwin GH, Grey RES, et al (1987) Effects of intravenous etidronate disodium on skeletal and calcium metabolism. Am J Med 82:55–70

Kofman S, Medrek TJ, Alexander RW (1964) Mithramycin in the treatment of embryonic cancer. Cancer 17:938–948

Krakoff IH, Newman RA, Goldberg RS (1979) Clinical toxicological and pharmacological studies of gallium nitrate. Cancer 44:1722–1727

Kuckla LJ, Abrahamson EC, McGyre WP, et al (1984) cis-Platinum treatment for malignancy-associated tumoral hypercalcemia in an athymic mouse model. Caclif Tissue Int 36:559–562

Lad TE, Mishoulam MH, Shevrin DH, et al (1987) Treatment of cancer-associated hypercalcemia with cis-platinum. Arch Intern Med 147:329–332

Lafferty FW (1966) Pseudohyperparathyroidism. Medicine (Baltimore) 45:247–260

Leow H, Wagner H (1973) Über den Wert der Hämodialyse-Therapie der hyperkalzämischen Krise beim primären Hyperparathyroidismus. Verh Dtsch Ges Inn Med 84:741

Lipton A (1996) Pamidronate and zelodronate: update on clinical results. Br J Clin Pract [Suppl] 87:21–22

Lipton A (1998) Zoledronate superior to pamidronate for bone metastases. Oncology News March–April:6

Miach PJ, Dawborne JK, Martin TJ (1975) Management of hypercalcemia of malignancy by peritoneal dialysis. Med J Aust 1:782–784

Monto RW, Talley RW, Caldwell MJ, et al (1969) Observations on the mechanism of hemorrhagic toxicity in mithramycin therapy. Cancer Res 29:697–704

Morton AR, Cantrill JA, Craig AE, et al (1988) Single dose versus daily intravenous amino-hydroxy-propylidene bisphosphonate (APD) for the hypercalcemia of malignancy. Br Med J 296:811–814

Mundy GR (1989) Calcium homeostasis, hypercalcemia and hypocalcemia: treatment of hypercalcemia due to malignancy. Dunitz, London, pp 108–126

Mundy GR (1990) Calcium homeostasis. Dunitz, London

Mundy GR, Martin TJ (1982) The hypercalcemia of malignancy: pathogenesis and management. Metabolism 31:1247–1277

Mundy GR, Kofe DH, Fisken R (1980) Primary hyperparathyroidism: changes in pattern of clinical presentation. Lancet 1:1317–1320

Mundy GR, Wilkinson R, Heath DA (1983) Comparative study of available medical therapy for hypercalcemia of malignancy. Am J Med 74:421–432

Nussbaum SR, Malette L, Gagel R, et al (1989) Single dose treatment of hypercalcemia of malignancy with aminohydroxypropylidene bisphosphonate (APD). J Bone Miner Res 4:313 (abstract)

Nussbaum SR, Warrell RP jr, Rude R, Glusman, et al (1993) Dose-response study of alendronate sodium for the treatment of cancer-associated hypercalcemia. J Clin Oncol 1:1918–1923

O'Rourke NP, McCloskey EV, Rosini S, Coleman RE, Kanis JA (1994) Treatment of malignant hypercalcemia with aminohexane bisphosphonate (neridronate). Br J Cancer 69:914–917

Pechersdorfer M, Hermann Z, Body JJ, Manegold C, Degardin M, Clemens RM, Thürlimann B, et al (1996) Randomized phase II trial comparing different doses of the bisphosphonate ibandronate in the treatment of hypercalcemia of malignancy. J Clin Oncol 14:268–276

Percival RC, Yates AJP, Gray RES (1984) The role of glucocorticoids in the management of malignant hypercalcaemia. Br Med J 290:289–287

Percival RC, Jates AJP, Grey RES, et al (1985) Mechanisms of hypercalcemia in carcinoma of the breast. Br Med J 291:776–779

Perlia CP, Gubisch NJ, Wolter J, et al (1970) Mithramycin treatment of hypercalcemia. Cancer 25:389–394

Plimpton CH, Gellhorn A (1956) Hypercalcemia in malignant disease without evidence of bone destruction. Am J Med 21:750–759

Proadus AE, Mangin M, Kyoji I, Insogna KL, Weir EC, Burtis WJ, Stewart AF (1988) Tumoral hypercalcemia of cancer: identification of a novel parathyroid hormone-like peptide. N Engl J Med 319:556–563

Ralston SH (1996) Ibandronate: a new therapeutic approach for the treatment of tumor-related bone disease; 3rd workshop on bisphosphonates, Davos, Switzerland, January 12, 1996

Ralston SH, Fogelman I, Gardner MD, Boyle IT (1984) Relative contribution of humeral and metastastic factors to the pathogenesis of hypercalcemia in malignancy. Br Med J 288:812–813

Ralston SH, Gardner MD, Dreiburg HFJ, Jenkins AS, Cowan RA, Boyle ET (1985) Comparison of aminohydroxypropylidene bisphosphonate, mithramycin and corticosteroids/calcitonin in the treatment of cancer-associated hypercalcemia. Lancet 2:907–910

Ralston SH, Fogelman I, Gardner MD, Boyle IT (1987) Hypercalcemia in metastatic bone disease: is there a causal link? Lancet 1:903–905

Ralston SH, Boyce BF, Cowan RH, Gardner ND, Fraser WD, Boyle IT (1989a) Contrasting mechanisms of hypercalcemia in patients with early and advanced humeral hypercalcemia of malignancy. J Bone Miner Res 4:103–111

Ralston SH, Patel U, Fraser WD, et al (1989b) Comparison of 3 intravenous bisphosphonates in cancer-associated hypercalcemia. Lancet 2:1180–1182

Ralston SH, Garacher SJ, Patel U, Cambel J, Boyle IT (1990) Cancer-associated hypercalcemia: morbidity and mortality experience in 126 patients. Ann Intern Med 112:499–504

Ralston SH, Thiébaud D, Herrmann Z, et al (1997) Dose-response study of ibandronate in treatment of cancer-associated hypercalcemia. Br J Cancer 75:295–300

Ringerberg QS, Ritch PS (1987) Efficacy of oral administration of etidronate in maintaining normal serum calcium levels in previously hypercalcemic cancer patients. Clin Ter 9:1-7

Ritch P, Gucalp R, Wiernik P, et al (1992) Pamidronate and EHDP in hypercalcemia of malignancy. J Clin Oncol 10:134-142

Rizzoli R, Buchs B, Bonjour JP (1992) Effect of a single infusion of alendronate in malignant hypercalcemia: dose dependency and comparison with clodronate. Int J Cancer 50:706-712

Senn HJ, Peyer P (1978) Die Therapie des Hypercalcämiesyndroms bei Tumorpatienten. Dtsch Med Wochenschr 103:101-107

Seyberth HW, Segre GV, Morgan JL, Sweetman BJ, Potts JT, Oates JA (1975) Prostaglandins as mediators of hypercalcemia in certain types of cancer. N Engl J Med 273:1278-1283

Sleeboom HP, Bijvoet OLM, van Oosteroom AT, Gleed JH, O'Reordan JLH (1983) Comparison of intravenous (3-amino-1-hydroxypropylidene)-1,1-bisphosphonate and volume repletion in tumor-induced hypercalcemia. Lancet 2:239-243

Strauch BS, Ball MF (1976) Hemodialysis in the treatment of severe hypercalcemia. JAMA 253:1347-1348

Stuart HF, Horst RL, Deftors LJ, Cadman EC, Lang R, Broadus AE (1980) Biochemical evaluation of patients with cancer-associated hypercalcemia: evidence for humeral and non-humeral groups. N Engl J Med 303:1377-1383

Suki WN, Yium JJ, Van Minden M, Saller-Hebert C, Eknoyan C, Martinez-Maldonato M (1970) Acute treatment of hypercalcemia with furosemide. N Engl J Med 283:836-840

Thalassinos N, Joplin GF (1970) Failure of corticosteroid therapy to correct the hypercalcaemia of malignant disease. Lancet 2:537-538

Thiébaud D, Jaeger PH, Jaquet AF, Burckardt P (1986a) A single day treatment of tumor-induced hypercalcemia by intravenous aminohydroypropylidene bisphosphonate. J Bone Miner Res 6:555-562

Thiébaud D, Portmann L, Jaeger PH, et al (1986b) Oral versus intravenous APD in the treatment of hypercalcemia of malignancy in bone. Bone 7:247-253

Thiébaud D, Jaeger P, Jacquet AF, et al (1988) Dose response in the treatment of hypercalcemia of malignancy by single infusion of the bisphosphonate AHPrBP (pamidronate). J Clin Oncol 6:762-768

Thürlimann B (1994) Progress in the treatment and palliation of advanced breast cancer: does the dose of pamidronate determine its effects? Ann Oncol 5:45-47

Thürlimann B, Waldburger R, Senn HJ, Thiébaud D (1992) Plicamycin and pamidronate in symptomatic tumor related hypercalcemia: a prospective randomised crossover trial. Ann Oncol 3:619-623

Warrell RP, Coonley CJ, Straus DJ, et al (1983) Treatment of patients with advanced malignant lymphoma using gallium nitrate administered as a seven day continuous infusion. Cancer 51:1982-1987

Warrell RP, Bockman RS, Coonely CJ, et al (1984) Gallium nitrate inhibits calcium resorption from bone and is effective treatment for cancer-related hypercalcemia. J Clin Invest 73:1487-1490

Warrell RP, Skelos A, Alcock NW, et al (1986) Gallium nitrate for acute treatment of cancer-related hypercalcemia: clinicopharmacological and dose response analysis. Cancer Res 46:4208-4212

Warrell RP, Alcock NW, Bockman RS (1987) Gallium nitrate inhibits accelerated bone turnover in patients with bone metastases. J Clin Oncol 5:292-298

Wisneski LA, Croom WP, Silva OL, Becker KL (1978) Calcitonin in hypercalcemia. Clin Pharmacol Ther 24:219-222

Wo G, Bonewald LF, Oreffo R, et al (1989) Evidence that lysosmal procathepsin D secreted by human breast cancer cells activates osteoclasts. J Bone Miner Res 5:S322 (abstract)

Wüster C, Schöter KH, Thiébaud D, et al (1993) Methylpentylaminopropylidene bisphosphonate (BM 21.0955): a new potent and safe bisphosphonate treatment of cancer-associated hypercalcemia. Bone Miner 22:77-85

Zondek H, Petow H, Siebert W (1924) Die Bedeutung der Calcium-Bestimmung im Blute für die Diagnose der Niereninsuffizienz. Z Klin Med 99:129-138

Malignant Osteolytic Bone Disease

Magnitude of the Problem

Radiological studies lead to antemortem diagnosis of bone metastases in about 50% of patients with metastatic cancer originating from breast, prostate, and lung cancer but in only 3–15% of patients with gastrointestinal tumors. According to autopsy series, 30–90% of patients with advanced cancer will develop skeletal metastases (Lote et al. 1986; Malaver and Delaney 1989). At the least, osteolytic bone disease can be responsible for considerable morbidity and a markedly decreased quality of life. Pain, pathological fractures, hypercalcemia, neurologic deficits, immobility, and side effects of analgesia, as well as anxiety and depression associated with complications of malignant osteolytic bone disease compromise the quality of the limited time remaining for these patients. This must be kept in mind whenever a treatment with palliative intention is being planned.

Metastasis is not an event but involves a number of highly selective steps, whereby in a subpopulation with adequate metastatic potential, which preexists in the primary tumor at the time of diagnosis or can develop later during treatment, it will spread via the blood stream to establish secondary deposits throughout the body. The steps in the pathogenesis of bone metastases are reviewed and described elsewhere (Sidler and Radinski 1990). In brief, these steps include invasion of the tumor into surrounding normal tissue, penetration of blood and lymphatic vessels, release of tumor cells into the circulation, attachment of tumor cells to the bone marrow, adherence to the endothelium, retraction of the endothelium, adhesion to the basement membrane, the dissolution of the basement membrane, and finally cell movement into the interstitial space. Having arrived there, the tumor cell has to create a favorable environment to ensure tumor cell survival, and to initiate replication and continuous tumor growth by neovascularization. Finally, these tumor deposits destroy bone via the cellular mechanisms of bone resorption as described in the previous chapter. The predilection of some tumors for certain sites in bone has been ascribed to the anatomic relationship between venous drainage of the primary site and the blood supply of bones that are common sites of metastases (Paterson 1987; Manishen et al. 1986). However, this is an oversimplification. Most metastatic sites in bone cannot be predicted based on anatomic considerations alone. Possible explanations of organ tropism include the following: (a) Organ-specific growth may be stimulated by local growth factors or hormones present in the bone or bone marrow. (b) Circulating tumor cells may build a metastatic deposit in bone marrow more than in other tissues, because endothelial cells of bone marrow sinusoids lack a basement membrane and may even have gaps between them that make the wall more penetrable for tumor cells (Perrettoni and Carter 1986). Circulating tumor cells may adhere preferentially to the endothelial luminal surface only in specific bones at certain localizations which may be mediated through organ-specific endothelial determination such as glycoproteins. (c) After adherence to the endothelium and possibly even retraction of the latter, tumor cells may respond to factors diffusing locally out of the bone which act chemotactically to attract the cells. Degradation products of normal bone resorption proved to be chemotactic for tumor cells in vitro and have also been described in the previous chapters (Lam et al. 1981; Manishen et al. 1986). These factors include, among others: collagen type 1 and collagen fragments, fibroblast growth factors, ILGF1, and TGF-β (Vinholes and Cooleman 1995). This situation might be most important during the late stages of metastatic bone disease, where osteoclasts disappear but osteolysis continues (Galasko 1982). Breast cancer cells also secrete factors that can inhibit proliferation of osteoblast-like cells and apparently increase their sensitivity to osteolytic agents (Body 1995). This might explain the phenomenon whereby, in certain tumors such as myeloma or breast cancer, relatively uniform multiple osteolytic bone lesions without a radiological appearance of blastic activity can be observed. However, bone histology often shows features of osteoblastic bone or even osteosclerosis (Paterson 1987). The above-mentioned features indicate that there is probably osteoblastic activity around so-called pure lytic lesions. This could also explain the pathogenesis of purely osteoblastic metastases, for example, from breast cancer. PTHrP appears to be produced by prostate cancer cells: recent immunohistochemical studies have found its presence in prostate tumors. Bone resorption is thus increased in patients with osteoblastic metastases from prostate cancer, as shown by biochemical markers. On the other hand, TGF-β is probably of crucial importance for the blastic reaction. It is produced in larger quantities by prostate cancer cells than by benign prostate cells, and the transition from benign prostate hyperplasia to cancer is associated with the induction of elevated TGF-β_1 production, which could be important in prostate cancer development and progression. The activation of TGF-β produced by the prostate or the bone tissue itself could be enhanced by prostate-specific antigen, which can also stimulate the proliferation of osteoblast-like cells by itself. Finally, bone morphogenetic proteins (BMPs) could also play a role in the osteoinductive properties of prostate cancer cells. BMPs are expressed by several prostate cancer cell lines, and, with the exception of BMP-5, they are more often expressed in patients with bone metastases than in those without.

Interdisciplinary Management

The management of patients with malignant osteolytic bone disease as regards surgery, radiotherapy, systemic endocrine and chemotherapy, as well as radioisotopes, has been reviewed elsewhere (Nielson et al. 1991; Body 1995). Treatment of neoplastic bone pain with an emphasis on analgetics has also recently been reviewed (Thürlimann and de Stoutz 1996). The following sections concentrate on treatment of malignant osteolytic bone disease with bisphosphonates.

Etidronate

Etidronate is effective in tumor-induced hypercalcemia. The effect on pain is unclear and a prospective, randomized, double-blind, placebo-controlled study concerning pain from bone metastases of prostate cancer showed that etidronate was ineffective for palliation of bone pain (Carey and Lippert 1988; Smith 1989). Etidronate was also shown to be ineffective in the prevention of bone complications due to multiple myeloma in a double-blind trial involving 173 patients (Belch et al. 1991).

Oral Formulations of Second- and Third-generation Bisphosphonates

Oral formulations of the bisphosphonates clodronate and pamidronate have been investigated. The first study using clodronate showed very encouraging results (Elomaa et al. 1987), and early results of a Dutch study were also promising (Van Holten et al. 1987).

Two further, large-scale studies of patients with breast cancer metastatic to the skeleton, one with clodronate (Paterson et al. 1993) and one with pamidronate (Van Holten-Verzantvoort et al. 1993), indicated that the prolonged administration of oral bisphosphonates can reduce the frequency of morbid skeletal events by 28% and 38%, respectively. A double-blind, randomized trial of clodronate, 1600 mg/day, against placebo was performed in 173 patients with breast cancer metastatic to bone. Among the clodronate-treated group, there was a significant reduction in the incidence of hypercalcemic episodes and vertebral fractures and in the rate of vertebral deformity. The combined rate of all morbid skeletal events was significantly reduced, but survial in the two groups was similar. The tolerance of clodronate was excellent (Paterson et al. 1993). On the other hand, a randomized, placebo-controlled trial of 350 patients with newly diagnosed myeloma who were given 2.4 g clodronate daily for 2 years also showed a significant reduction in the proportion of patients presenting a progression of osteolytic bone lesions, from 24% to 12%, in an intention-to-treat analysis, although the progression rate of vertebral fractures was not significantly different between the two groups (Lahtinen et al. 1992). Despite these encouraging results, the place of oral bisphosphonates remains unclear, in the opinion of many clinicians. Furthermore, there is a considerable publication bias toward studies performed with oral clodronate.

The main drawback to the oral administration of bisphosponates is the fact that the absorption of available compounds is poor and variable, as discussed in the previous sections. The mean bioavailability of a 300-mg oral dose of pamidronate has been estimated to be around 0.3% (Daley-Yates et al. 1991). A similarly low figure of 0.5% has been reported for alendronate. The requirement to take the drug around 2 h before or after food intake, the occasional intolerance superimposed on the frequent digestive complaints or appetite of cancer patients, and the need for doses of bisphosphonates much higher in malignant osteolytic bone disease than in benign conditions make the intravenous route more attractive than the oral route, at least for cancer patients. However, this could change in the future, with newly developed third-generation compounds such as ibandronate or zoledronate. In a dose of 20 mg daily for 4 weeks, oral ibandronate was as effective in the reduction of bone turnover – measured by urinary calcium creatinine ratio and urinary pyridinoline and desoxipyridinoline excretion – as 2 mg ibandronate given intravenously in patients with osteolytic metastases of breast cancer (Boehringer Mannheim, data on file). These third-generation bisphosphonates in today's oral formulations are usually well tolerated but can rarely cause unpredictable severe toxicity. Ibandronate can rarely cause severe mucosal esophagitis and diarrhea (Boehringer Mannheim, data on file). Alendronate is reported to cause severe ulcerating esophagitis, which was observed not only as "pill esophagitis" but also as ulceration involving the esophagus in its entire length (de Groen et al. 1996; Liberman and Hirsch 1995). Post-marketing data through March 1996 include reports of adverse events related to the esophagus in 199 patients. Fifty-one of these were considered to have severe adverse effects of alendronate, and 32 had to be hospitalized (Castell 1996). It remains to be proven whether better formulation of oral bisphosphonates may help to reduce the risk of severe mucosal toxicity.

The aforementioned reasons and the need for rapid and effective palliation in patients with painful osteolytic bone disease led us to investigate the effects of pamidronate administered as an intravenous infusion. In the late 1980s the pharmacokinetics of pamidronate in cancer patients was unknown. There was an urgent need to reduce the usual infusion time of 24 h when 60 or 90 mg pamidronate was administered for osteolytic bone disease. A reduction of the infusion time to 4 h and if possible to an even a shorter time of 2 or 1 h was intended. Furthermore, there was a need to determine the influence of the infusion rate on bone turnover. Up to then it was believed that prolonged infusion would be more effective than a shorter infusion because saturation of the skeleton would be higher the longer the exposure of bisphosphonates to the bone surface. This hypothesis was based on limited pharmacokinetic data concerning clodronate in healthy subjects, where means of 73% and 81% of the administered dose of clodronate were found unchanged in the urine within 24 and 48 h, respectively, with no difference between three doses tested (Conrad and Lee 1981; Jakathan et al. 1982). In six patients with metastatic breast cancer total urinary excretion of clodronate was found to be similar at 75% (Pentikäinen et al. 1989). In patients with Paget's disease mean urine excretion was lower, at 58%, because clodronate was administered as daily intervenous infusions for 5 consecutive days. It was concluded that slow infusions would increase accumulation in the body and possibly in bone (Hanhijärvi et al. 1989).

References

Belch AR, Bergsagel DE, Wilson K, et al (1991) Effect of daily etidronate on the osteolysis of multiple myeloma. J Clin Oncol 9:1397–1402

Body JJ (1995) Bone metastases. In: Klastersky J, Schimpff SC, Senn HJ (eds) Handbook of supportive care in cancer. Dekker, New York, pp 365–401

Carey PO, Lippert MC (1988) Treatment of pain for prostatic bone metastasis with oral etidronate disodium. Urology 32:403–407

Castell OD (1996) Pill esophagitis – the case of alendronate. N Engl J Med 35:1058–1059

Conrad KA, Lee SM (1981) Clodronate: kinetics and dynamics. Clin Pharmacol Ther 30:114–120

Daley-Yates PT, Dodwell DJ, Pongchaidecha M, Coleman RE, Howell A (1991) The clearance and bioavailability of pamidronate in patients with breast cancer and bone metastases. Calcif Tissue Int 49:433–435

de Groen PC, Lubbe DF, Hirsch LS, et al (1996) Oesophagitis associated with the use of alendronate. N Engl J Med 35:1016–1021

Elomaa I, Blomquist C, Porkka L, Lamberg-Allard D, Bergström GH (1987) Treatment of skeletal disease in breast cancer: a controlled clodronate trial. Bone 8:56–58

Galasko CSB (1982) Mechanisms of lytic and blastic metastatic disease of bone. Clin Orthop 169:20–27

Hanhijärvi H, Elomaa I, Carlson M, et al (1989) Pharmacokinetics of disodium clodronate after daily intravenous infusions during 5 consecutive days. Int J Clin Pharmacol Ther Toxicol 27:602–606

Jakathan GI, Poynor WI, Thalbert RL, et al (1982) Clodronate: kinetics and bioavailability. Clin Pharmacol Ther 31:402–410

Lahtinen R, Laakso M, Palva I, Virkkunen P, Elomaa I (1992) Finnish Leukemia Group. Randomized placebo-controlled multicenter trial of clodronate in multiple myeloma. Lancet 340:1049–1052

Lam WC, Delicathny EJ, Or FW, et al (1981) The chemotactic response of tumor cells: a model for cancer metastasis. Am J Pathol 104:69–76

Liberman UA, Hirsch LJ (1995) Esophagitis and alendronate. N Engl J Med 33:1069–1070

Lote K, Vallue A, Bjersand A (1986) Bone metastasis. Prognosis, diagnosis and treatment. Acta Radiol Oncol 25:227–232

Malaver MM, Delaney TF (1989) Treatment of metastatic cancer to bone. In: De Vita VT, Hellman S, Rosenberg SA (eds) Cancer, principles and practise of oncology. Lippincott, Philadelphia, pp 2298–2317

Manishen WJ, Swinanthan K, Orr FW (1986) Resorbing bone stimulates tumor cell growth. Am J Pathol 123:39–45

Nielson OS, Munrow AJ, Tannock IF (1991) Bone metastasis: pathophysiology and management policy. J Clin Oncol 9:509–524

Paterson AHG (1987) Bone metastases in breast cancer, prostate cancer and myeloma. Bone 8:17–22

Paterson AHG, Powles TJ, Kanis JA, McCloskey E, Hanson J, Ashley S (1993) Double-blind controlled trial of oral clodronate in patients with bone metastases from breast cancer. J Clin Oncol 11:59–65

Pentikäinen PJ, Elomaa I, Nurmi KH, et al (1989) Pharmacokinetics of clodronate in patients with metastatic breast cancer. Int J Clin Pharmacol Ther Toxicol 27:222–228

Perrettoni BA, Carter JR (1986) Mechanisms of cancer metastasis to bone. J Bone Joint Surg 86A:308–312

Sidler IJ, Radinski R (1990) Genetic control of cancer metastases. J Natl Cancer Inst 82:166–168

Smith JA (1989) Palliation of painful bone metastases from prostate cancer using disodium etidronate: results of a randomised prospective double-blind placebo-controlled study. J Urol 141:85–87

Thürlimann B, de Stoutz N (1996) Causes and treatment of bone pain of malignant origin – disease managment. Drugs 51:383–398
Van Holten A, Bijvoet OLM, Cleaton FJ (1987) Reduced morbidity from skeletal metastases in breast cancer patients during long-term bisphosphonate (APD) treatment. Lancet 2:983–985
Van Holton-Verzantvoort ATM, Kroon HM, Bijvoet OLM, et al (1993) Palliative pamidronate treatment in patients with bone metastases from breast cancer. J Clin Oncol 11:491–498
Vinholes J, Cooleman R (1995) The management of bone metastasis. Ann Oncol 6:713–720

Pamidronate

Pharmacokinetics of Pamidronate in Patients with Bone Metastases (SG 121/89, internal protocol number)

Because of the need to shorten infusion time for reasons of practicability, and because it was not known to what extent the pharmacokinetics of pamidronate might be affected by the rate of administration, a prospective pharmacokinetic study of pamidronate at three different infusion rates was started in the Department of Internal Medicine C, Kantonsspital St. Gallen KSSG, Switzerland and in the Centre Pluridisciplinaire d'Oncologie and the Department of Internal Medicine, both at the University Hospital in Lausanne CHUV, Switzerland. A total of 37 patients with bone metastases were included in the study and treated in three groups of 11–14 patients each. Pamidronate was administered as an intravenous infusion of 60 mg over a period of 1, 4, or 24 h. All patients had serum creatinine levels less than 150 µmol/l, and none of the patients had been treated previously with bisphosphonates. No new medication and no chemotherapy was started for at least 72 h prior to entry or at any time during the study. Median creatinine clearance was 66 ml/min (range 37–110 ml/min). Mean age was 63 years (range 28–78 years). Thirty-two of the 37 patients suffered from bone metastases of breast cancer. The study was performed in two phases over a 15-month period. During the first phase, 23 patients were randomly assigned to receive 60 mg pamidronate as a 4-h or a 24-h infusion. Patients had an additional 2 l of intravenous fluid intake during the day of pamidronate administration as well as on the following day. When analysis disclosed that the amount of the drug excreted in the urine was similar at both infusion rates, the second phase of the study was started with an additional 14 patients. They received 60 mg pamidronate in 250 ml 0.9% NaCl solution over a period of 1 h without hydration. In this group of patients not only urine samples but also blood samples were collected. Four of the 14 patients in the second group were selected to receive repeated 1-h infusions at 4- to 5-week intervals for a maximum of four infusions. In all patients toxicity was closely monitored, especially renal toxicity. Serum urea, creatinine, calcium, phosphate, albumin, bilirubin, alkaline phosphatase, and transaminases were checked daily. In addition, calcium, phosphate, creatinine, sodium, hydroxyproline, and lysozyme were examined in the urine. Clinical monitoring for toxicity was performed daily during the infusion period and then after 2 and after 4 weeks. In all patients the number of bone metastases was evaluated on standard X-rays. The assay of pamidronate in plasma and urine was performed with high-performance liquid chromatography. The original hypothesis that the faster the infusion, the greater the loss of bisphosphonate in the urine was not confirmed. On the contrary, the total 24-h urinary excretion of pamidronate was not significantly different and was measured at 31%±15.2%, 34.9%±13.9%, and 41.0%±15.4% of the 60 mg of pamidronate infused over 1 h, 4 h, and 24 h, respectively. Considerable interpatient variability was observed, as expected. Twenty-four-hour urinary excretion was correlated with creatinine clearance and with the extent of metastatic bone involvment. Only a weak relationship was observed as analyzed by linear chi-square regression ($r=0.42$), but a stronger association was seen between numbers of bone metastases and 24-h body retention. Further details of the study are reported elsewhere (Hess et al. 1991; Leyvraz et al. 1992).

References

Hess U, Senn HJ, Ford J, et al (1991) Influence of infusion rate on pharmacokinetics of intravenous pamidronate (APD) in patients with bone metastases. In: Bijvoet O (ed) Proceedings of the international symposium on osteoclast inhibition in the management of malignancy-related bone disorders, Hamburg

Leyvraz S, Hess U, Flesh G, et al (1992) Pharmacokinectics of pamidronate in patients with bone metastases. J Natl Cancer Inst 84:788–792

Pamidronate for Pain Control in Patients with Malignant Osteolytic Bone Disease: A Prospective Dose-Effect Study (SG 88/90)

Having established a safer and more convenient schedule for administering pamidronate in doses which were known to induce pain relief (Hacking et al. 1991), we investigated the safety of repeated infusions of high doses of pamidronate and correlated dose intensity with palliative effect.

Patients and Methods

A group of 80 patients with proven malignancy and pain due to osteolytic bone disease were enrolled. Inclusion criteria required at least one painful lesion outside a radiation field if the patient was receiving radiotherapy. Serum creatinine had to be no more than 350 mmol/l. Hemoglobin, white cells and platelets, creatinine, and calcium were determined before each infusion.

Table 3. Patient and treatment characteristics

Characteristic	No.
Patient number, total	80
Diagnosis	
Breast cancer	39
Myeloma	26
Other tumors	15
Infusions given, total	419
Dose time intervals	88
In patients with progressive disease	68
In patients without progressive disease	20
Infusions given in evaluable patients	390
Mean no. of infusions per patient	4.43
Range	2–44
Cumulative dose (mg)	
Mean	281
Range	60–1305

The trial began with 30 mg pamidronate given intravenously every 4 weeks. The dose was subsequently increased, both in patients already on treatment and in those newly enrolled, by giving 30 mg every 3 weeks, followed by 30 mg every 2 weeks if pain control was unsatisfactory – as rated by the treating physician on a six-point scale. Higher doses of 45 mg, 60 mg, and 90 mg pamidronate every 4, 3, or 2 weeks were also evaluated, corresponding to 12 intended doses. Dose intensity was thus increased by giving higher single doses and/ or by shortening the intervals. Pamidronate was usually given in 500 ml 0.9% NaCl as an intravenous infusion over 1–2 h, but in patients with serum creatinine at or above 180 mmol/l the drug was administered over 4–8 h.

Treatment was given on an outpatient basis. Most patients had breast cancer or myeloma and had progressive disease with poor performance status. Additional treatment for the underlying malignant disease was allowed and documented; all patients were receiving regular analgesics at study entry. Patient characteristics are summarized in Table 3.

Results

A total of 419 infusions were administered. Documentation was inadequate on five patients. At 88 intended dose time intervals more than one infusion was given, and the dose intensity of all given infusions at the actual times was calculated. These patients received a total of 390 infusions (mean 4.43, range 2–44). The mean cumulative pamidronate dose was 281 mg (range 60–1305 mg). Sixty-eight of the patients receiving two or more infusions had progressive disease. Twenty patients had no change or partial remission.

Efficacy was assessed on the basis of pain score (WHO criteria), analgesic score (WHO criteria), and improvement of performance status (SAKK/ ECOG). A combined palliation score, calculated on the basis of the above-mentioned parameters, was rated by the physician on a six-point scale, ranging from zero (no effect) to 5 (excellent effect) at the time of best response.

Statistical analysis was performed using regression analysis and parametric and nonparametric comparisons as required.

In patients who received pamidronate at the lower dosage and at infrequent intervals, clinically significant effects were rarely observed. Single doses of 30 mg usually effected no relevant pain relief. With higher doses there was a clear palliative effect, however: 90 mg pamidronate had a beneficial effect in most patients, especially if given every 3 or every 2 weeks.

Regression analysis showed a close correlation between dose intensity and effect, as expressed by the palliative score (Pearson's $r=0.7$, $p=0.0001$). The coefficient for the slope of the curve ($y=0.1x+0.372$) was 0.1 ± 0.011 (Fig. 4). The same dose-effect relationship was shown by forming and comparing treatment groups of low (up to 15 mg/week), medium (16–30 mg/week), and high dose (above 31 mg pamidronate per week) intensity. The differences in the mean palliative scores at the three dose levels (0.13 versus 3.0 versus 4.2) were statistically significant (Wilcoxon signed-rank test: $p<0.01$). A dose intensity below 10 mg pamidronate per week showed no clinically relevant benefit, whereas dose intensities of 20–45 mg/week had a significant palliative effect (see Fig. 5). Many patients treated at high dose intensity showed a striking improvement in their condition and refused to stop treatment or decrease the dose. There was no significant difference in the slope of the linear regression curve for patients with breast cancer, myeloma, or other malignant tumors. Regression analysis showed a statistically significant dose-effect relationship, both for patients with progressive disease in spite of antineoplastic systemic therapy

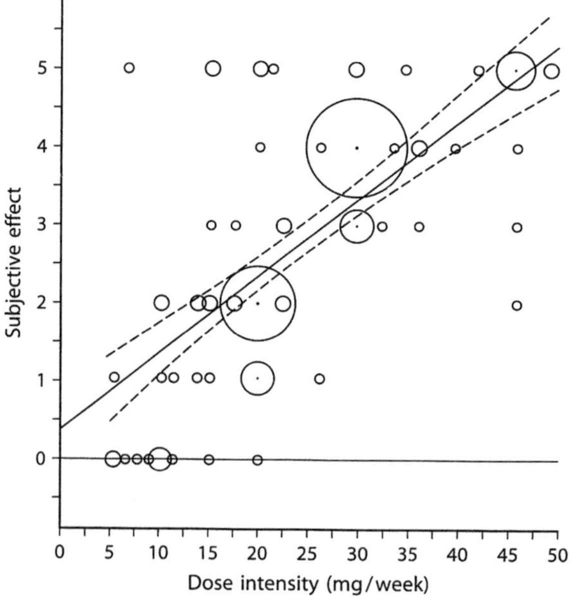

Fig. 4. Pamidronate: linear correlation of dose intensity and palliative effect rated by the treating physician (±90% CI). Dot size reflects number of patients (smallest dots represent one patient, largest dot 12 patients)

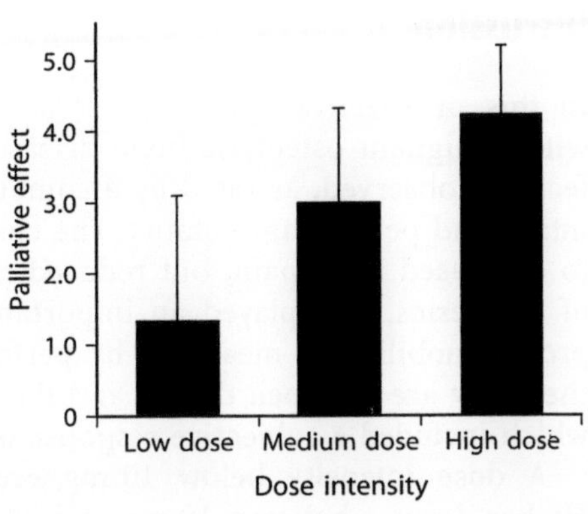

Fig. 5. Mean palliative scores in treatment groups: low dose (up to 15 mg APD per week, $n=19$); medium dose (16–30 mg APD per week, $n=44$); high dose (>31 mg APD per week, $n=18$). *Error bars* standard error. Differences between means are statistically highly significant ($p<0.001$, Wilcoxon signed rank test)

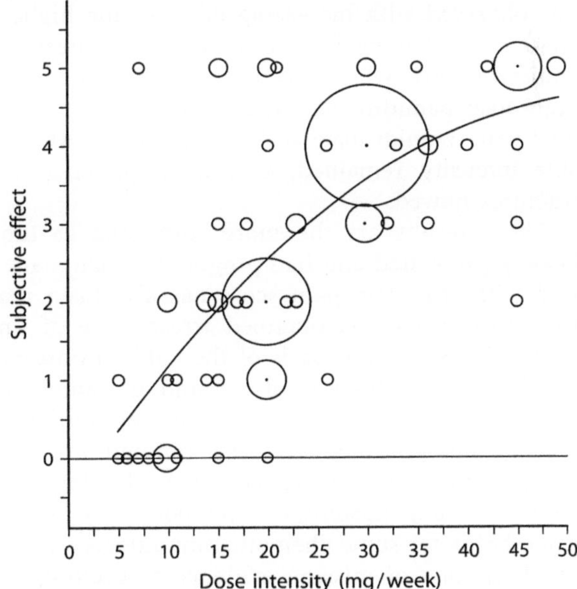

Fig. 6. Pamidronate: second-grade polynominal correlation of dose intensity and subjective, palliative effect as rated by the physician (±90% CI). Dot size reflects number of patients (smallest dots represent one patient, largest dot 12 patients)

($n=67$; $y=0.102x+0.136$, $r=0.493$, $p=0.0001$) and for patients whose tumor either was stable or responded to concomitant systemic therapy ($n=20$; $y=0.075x+1.681$, $r=0.39$, $p=0.005$). The mean palliative score, however, was significantly higher in patients without progressive disease than in those with progressive disease (mean palliative score 3.7 versus 2.5 with standard errors of 0.317 and 0.202; Mann-Whitney test: $p=0.007$).

As shown in a secondary polynomial regression-analysis curve (Fig. 6), the dose-effect relationship curve flattens out at higher doses.

No clinically relevant toxicity was seen, except in two myeloma patients with preexisting elevated serum creatinine in whom the serum creatinine further increased.

Discussion

In this prospective open dose-escalation study of pamidronate in patients with malignant osteolytic bone disease, a clear dose-dependant palliative effect was observed, as rated by a combined score based on pain and analgesic intake and performance status. The change in palliative score was due mainly to decreased bone pain, but reduced analgesic intake, with fewer side effects of analgesics, also played an important role. Most patients also showed improved mobility, as measured by performance status. Possible weaknesses of the study are the open design and the method of judging the palliative score, which included a subjective response of the physician involved.

A dose intensity below 10 mg/week had no clinically relevant benefit. Higher doses – between 10 mg and 20 mg/week – showed some effect, but in patients treated with between 20 mg and 40 mg/week a pronounced effect was observed with increasing dose. At the highest dose intensities the dose-effect curve flattened again, as may be expected by the construction of the palliative score, which has a maximum value of 5. Most patients treated with high-dose pamidronate experienced excellent palliation. In those with residual pain, pamidronate at 45 mg/week was usually effective, but pain of variable intensity remained, e.g., when patients with preexisting pathological fractures moved.

These results are the more surprising as the majority of patients were heavily pretreated and had progressive malignant disease. The same observation with regard to pain score has also been made also by other investigators. Pain relief was obtained irrespective of final outcome (Morton et al. 1989). The biological basis of the baffling observation that a subjective effect of bisphosphonates was also found in radiologically progressive disease is unknown, and explanations would be purely speculative: apparently, the mechanisms of tumor osteolysis and pain are not necessarily interwoven and can in some situations be separated. This important finding stresses the relevance of using meaningful end points to judge medical interventions. The same holds for some chemotherapy interventions, when palliation may be offered in spite of missing evidence of prolonged survival or even tumor regression.

The regression lines for patients with responding or stable disease were less steep and did not cross the zero point (intercept coefficient 1.6), in contrast to those for patients with progressive disease (intercept coefficient 0.1). This interesting observation is most probably explained by the analgesic effect of successful chemotherapy for the underlying malignant disease. As expected, these patients experienced pain relief at very low doses of pamidronate, even at dose intensity "zero", showing the palliative effect of efficient chemotherapy for the underlying disease (Fig. 7). Therefore, the mean change on the six-point palliation scale was greater in the patient group without progressive disease compared with that in patients with progressive underlying malignant disease. However, this observation is due mainly to the effect in patients treated at lower dose intensity (and with successful che-

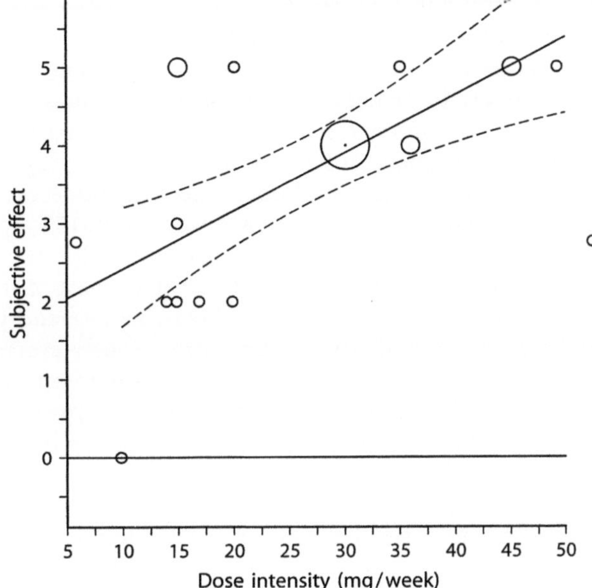

Fig. 7. Pamidronate: linear correlation of dose intensity and palliative effect as rated by treating physician (±90% CI), patients with nonprogressive disease only ($n = 20$). Dot size reflects number of patients (smallest dots represent one patient, largest dot five patients)

motherapy). The regression lines converge with higher dose intensity, and confidence intervals overlap in patients treated with at least 30 mg pamidronate per week. This observation may well indicate that selected patients with a fair chance of response to antineoplastic therapy can be treated with lower doses of pamidronate and still achieve satisfactory palliation. The selection of a patient population which will benefit most from pamidronate treatment remains a challenge, as the results of this study showed no significant differences in the dose-effect curves for patients with different diagnoses. However, a conclusion can be drawn only for patients with breast cancer and myeloma, because the number of patients with identical diagnoses in the subgroup "other diagnosis" was too low.

No clinically relevant toxicity was observed. Two patients with myeloma and preexisting elevated creatinine levels showed a further increase after the first pamidronate infusion. These changes in serum creatinine might reflect either a real side effect of pamidronate or a state of altered hydration at the time of creatinine analysis, as frequently seen in advanced myeloma and impaired kidney function. In one patient the serum creatinine returned to the preexisting level, and treatment with a longer infusion time was continued. In the second patient, serum creatinine declined, but treatment was stopped after the first infusion, because the return was not to the pretreatment level.

The results seen in our study compare well with the experience of other investigators using bisphosphonates as an analgesic treatment for patients with osteolytic bone disease. Oral and intravenous clodronate has shown a clear analgesic effect compared with placebo (Delmas et al. 1982; Elomaa et al. 1987; Paterson et al. 1991). Oral pamidronate has also demonstrated a significant analgesic effect and a decrease in bone-associated complications compared with the control in a prospective randomized trial (Van Holten et al. 1987).

A single infusion of 90 mg pamidronate had a significant palliative effect in terminally ill breast cancer patients without antineoplastic treatment. This effect was sustained for 3–4 weeks in most patients (Hacking et al. 1991). Single pamidronate infusions at doses ranging from 15 mg to 120 mg achieved a prolonged inhibitory effect on bone breakdown, as measured by urinary calcium excretion: high doses of 90–120 mg pamidronate were more effective than doses of 15–60 mg (Body 1992).

The dose and schedule of pamidronate have also been investigated in an American study in patients with breast cancer and prostate cancer. As in our study, 30 mg pamidronate given intravenously every 4 weeks had no measurable effect either subjectively, concerning pain and other parameters of quality of life, or objectively, in reducing bone resorption (Lipton et al. 1992). When the dose intensity was increased, partly by shortening the interval between infusions but mainly by increasing the dose, a significant improvement of pain relief was observed. The analgesic score decreased also, but only in patients treated with 60 mg or 90 mg pamidronate. Improvement in symptoms other than pain and performance status (as seen in our study) was also observed in a study of breast cancer patients treated with high-dose intravenous pamidronate (30 mg weekly for 4 weeks, followed by bi-weekly administration) (Morton et al. 1989). Another investigation showed that intrapatient dose escalation resulted in a clear palliative effect for patients in whom pain control was unsatisfactory with low-dose treatment (Radziwill et al. 1993).

In this study, objective tumor response, as indicated by sclerosis of lytic lesions before start of pamidronate treatment, was seen in about a quarter of the patients (Bacchus and Thürlimann 1994). This observation corresponds well to the above-mentioned American phase-II study of 60 patients with progressive metastatic bone disease due to breast cancer using 30 and 60 mg pamidronate every 2 weeks or 60 and 90 mg pamidronate very 4 weeks. In this study no patient received either systemic antineoplastic treatment or radiotherapy. In 25% of patients radiographic changes consistent with remineralization of lytic skeletal lesions were noted, while stabilization was obtained in a other 47% (Grabelsky et al. 1991). Three smaller studies showed evidence of sclerosis in about a quarter of the patients with previously lytic lesions (Cooleman et al. 1988; Morton et al. 1988; Burckardt et al. 1989). In one study evidence of sclerosis of lytic metastases was seen in four of 16 patients and disease stabilization in four others. Concentration of both carcinoembryonic antigen and carbohydrate antigen CA 15–3 decreased in three patients (two had partial response and one disease stabilization), remained unchanged in eight, and increased in five. Patients who showed radiological improvement tended to have a particularly low urinary calcium creatinine ratio after the first infusion. On the other hand, patients' perception of their pain, expressed as a percentage on a linear analogue scale, decreased significantly but was unrelated to radiological response (Morton et al. 1989).

Conclusion

When the data from dose-seeking studies are pooled, it appears that clear relief of bone pain can be obtained in more than one of three patients and objective sclerosis of the lytic lesions in one of four patients. Pamidronate infusions given at doses greater than 15 mg/week are necessary for significant relief of pain associated with malignant osteolytic bone disease. A dose intensity of less than 15 mg/week and single doses of 30 mg or less are not effective. Pamidronate should be given at a dose intensity of 20 mg/week or more. Best results, with early relief of pain, are obtained with high doses of 60 mg or 90 mg pamidronate, as shown by the two dose-escalation studies of Lipton and co-workers and Thürlimann and co-workers. Loading doses followed by lower doses of pamidronate, as investigated by a British group, may also be a successful strategy. Further investigations in prospective randomized trials to determine the optimal dose and schedule are needed.

References

Bacchus L, Thürlimann B (1994) Remineralisation of osteolytic malignant bone disease after repeated pamidronate infusions: a retrospective analysis. Ann Oncol 5:213 (abstract)

Body JJ (1992) Pamidronate for tumor-induced hypercalcaemia and tumor-induced osteolyses: what is the optimal therapeutic regimen? Proc Am Soc Clin Oncol 11:411 (abstract)

Burckardt P, Thiébaud D, Perey L, Von Fliedner V (1989) Treatment of tumor-induced osteolysis by APD. In: Herfarth C, Senn HJ (eds) Recent results in cancer research, vol 116. Springer, Berlin Heidelberg New York, pp 54–66

Cooleman R, Wol PJ, Miles M, Screvener W, Rubens RD (1988) 3-Amino-1,1-hydroxypropyledene bisphosphonate (APD) for the treatment of bone metastasis from breast cancer. Br J Cancer 58:621

Delmas PD, Charhorn S, Chapuy MC, Vignon E, Briançon D (1982) Long-term effects of dichloromethylene disphosphonate (Cl_2MDP) on skeletal lesions in muliple myeloma. Metab Bone Dis Relat Res 4:163–168

Elomaa I, Blomquist C, Porkka L, Lamberg-Allard D, Bergström GH (1987) Treatment of skeletal disease in breast cancer: a controlled clodronate trial. Bone 8:53–56

Grabelsky S, Lipton A, Harvey H, et al (1991) Pamidronate disodium (APD), a dose seeking study in patients with breast cancer. Proc Am Soc Clin Oncol 10:42 (abstract)

Hacking A, Gudgeon CA, Mac Naughton D, Dent DM (1991) Pamidronate (APD) as single infusion monotherapy in the treatment of bone metastases from breast cancer. In: Bijvoet OLM, Lipton A (eds) Osteoclast inhibition in the management of malignancy-related bone disorders. Hogrefe and Huber, Lewingston, pp 45–53

Lipton A, Grobelsky S, Glover D, Harvey H, Simone J, Seaman J (1992) Pamidronate disodium (APD): the American experience in breast and prostate cancer. Bone Miner 17:27 (abstract)

Morton A, Dodwell DJ, Howell A (1989) Disodium pamidronate APD infusions for bone metastases: clinical trial in patients with breast carcinoma. In: Burkardt P (ed) Disodium pamidronate (APD) in the treatment of malignancy-related disorders. Huber, Toronto, pp 120–133

Morton AR, Cantrill JA, Pillai GV, McMahon A, Anderson DC, Howell H (1988) Sclerosis of lytic bone metastasis after disodium aminohydroxypropyledene bisphosphonate (APD) in patients with breast cancer. Br Med J 297:772–773

Paterson AHG, Ernst DS, Powels TJ, Ashley S, Mc Closkey EV, Kamis JA (1991) Treatment of skeletal disease in breast cancer with clodronate. Bone 12:25–30
Radziwill AJ, Thürlimann B, Jungi WF (1993) Improvement of palliation in patients with osteolytic bone disease and unsatisfactory pain control after pretreatment with disodium pamidronate: an intrapatient dose escalation study. Onkologie 16:174–177
Van Holten A, Bijvoet OLM, Cleaton FJ (1987) Reduced morbidity from skeletal metastases in breast cancer patients during long-term bisphosphonate (APD) treatment. Lancet 2:983–985

A Prospective, Randomized, Dose-finding Study of Pamidronate in Patients with Malignant Osteolytic Bone Disease (SG 99/91)

Having established a safe and more practical mode of repeated administration, and having analyzed the data of our dose-escalation study and the study performed by A. Lipton and co-workers, we started a prospective randomized study of patients with malignant osteolytic bone disease and pain. This was conceived as an original multicenter study involving patients from several regional hospitals, from a private oncologist, and from the Department of Internal Medicine C, Division Oncology/Hematology of the Kantonsspital St. Gallen. The aim of the study was to compare the palliative effect of 60 mg pamidronate versus 90 mg pamidronate administered intravenously every 3 weeks.

Patients and Methods

Eligibility criteria included histologically or cytologically proven malignancy and osteolytic bone metastases or primary osteolytic bone involvement (e.g., multiple myeloma) and pain (WHO pain score >2), irrespective of prior antineoplastic treatment. Approval of the local hospital ethical committee was obtained, as well as informed consent from all patients. All other treatments which were regarded as being in the best interest of the patients were allowed and had to be documented. Exclusion criteria were bisphosphonate exposure within 4 weeks before study entry (and throughout the whole study with exception of the trial medication), serum creatinine >240 µmol/l, concomitant hormonal therapy, pregnancy/lactation, terminal status of the patient. Following stratification for diagnosis, the patients were randomized centrally by prepared envelopes. Between November 1991 and October 1992, 50 patients were enrolled over a period of 11 months by the Department of Internal Medicine C, Division Oncology/Hematology. Patients were randomized to receive either 60 mg or 90 mg pamidronate intravenously in 250 ml NaCl 0.9% as an infusion given over 2 h and repeated every 3 weeks for a total of six infusions. The drug was supplied by Novartis, formerly Ciba Geigy Pharma Switzerland. No dose modifications were prescribed. Patient evaluation was performed at baseline (before starting therapy and thereafter before each infusion). Efficacy of antitumor therapy was evaluated according to WHO criteria. Performance status was assessed according to Swiss Group for Clinical Cancer Research (SAKK)/Eastern Cooperative Oncology Group (ECOG) criteria. The use of analgesic medication was recorded and categorized using a modified WHO analgesic score: none = 0, mild analgesics (e.g., paracetamol, acetylsalicylate) = 1, nonsteroidal anti-inflammatory drugs (e.g., diclofenac, ibuprofen) = 2, opioids (e.g., tramadol, codein) = 3, opiates (e.g., morphin, buprenorphin) = 4. When analgesics of more than one category were used, the highest category was assigned. Pain score (PSC) was assessed according to WHO criteria.

Subjective therapeutic efficacy of pamidronate was assessed using self-administered linear analogue scales (LASA) for pain intensity (PIN), pain frequency (PF), well-being (WB), and pain improvement (PIM) prior to each infusion.

Additionally, patients were asked: Do you believe that you benefit from the infusions? Answer categories were yes, no, I don't know.

Additional efficacy parameters were laboratory values: alkaline phosphatase (AP), osteocalcin (OST), serum calcium (SCA), and urinary calcium creatinine ratio in the second morning spot urine. Safety parameters were serum creatinine and serum calcium. Toxicity of the infusion was reported in a descriptive way.

Statistical Analysis

The study was planned to test the difference of change in pain intensity after three infusions between patients treated with pamidronate 60 mg and those who received 90 mg. It was estimated that the mean value of pain intensity at the baseline would be 0.60 in the linear analogue self-assessment LASA. We hypothesized that 60 mg pamidronate would reduce pain intensity by 20% (e.g., from 0.60 to 0.48), whereas pain intensity in the 90 mg arm would be reduced by 30% after three infusions had been administered (e.g., from 0.6 to 0.42 in the LASA scale). Thus, we were searching for a 50% difference in treatment efficacy regarding percent reduction of pain intensity after three infusions of pamidronate. To find this clinically relevant difference with a power of 80% we required a minimal sample size of 24 evaluable patients, 12 patients per treatment arm. The main analysis focused on the comparison of the two arms in terms of LASA scales, LAB values, and physician-rated SAKK/ECOG performance status (PS) and WHO pain score (PSC). Analysis was performed on an intention-to-treat basis.

The chi-square and Fisher's exact test were used for contingency tables. Baseline properties of PSC and LASA scales were investigated as follows: LASA scale correlation was analyzed using the Spearman rank correlation method, and a test for linear trend was used to compare the physician-rated pain score (PSC) and the patient-rated pain intensity (Cuzick 1995).

The Wilcoxon rank-sum test was used for ordered categorical tables. In general, changes in longitudinal data in the presence of missing values are difficult to analyze. With regard to the present data, only few patients had a complete set of assessments. As an alternative to repeated measure analysis (which requires complete and normally distributed data sets), we defined summary measures (Bernhard et al. 1996). Different summary measures of longitudinal assessment (LASA scores and LAB values) results are presented:

1. Overall mean: mean value of all assessments
2. Overall improvement: difference between baseline score (or value) and the average score (or value) recorded at subsequent visits (Robertson et al. 1995). The Wilcoxon signed-rank test was used to test the hypothesis of a zero difference from baseline. The Wilcoxon rank-sum test was used to compare the two arms.
3. Improvement in percent: difference between baseline score and the score recorded at subsequent visits (after first and third infusion) as percentage of the basline score. For categorical scales (PS; PSC, and use of analgesics) we defined an overall "increase"/"decrease" comparing baseline with the maximal category of subsequent visits. For example: an "increase" in analgesic use is attributed if the baseline analgesic is lower than the maximal analgesic category during pamidronate treatment. These summary measures were compared between treatments, and conclusions were reached only when consistency among results was seen.

The impact of pamidronate treatment on the summary measures was investigated with muliple regression analyses adjusted for baseline scores and selected covariates (Neter et al. 1985).

Graphical representations of LASA and LAB patterns over time were used descriptively (Hopwood et al. 1994). No paired comparison was performed because of different patients contributing data at each assessment point. Treatment duration (TD) was measured from randomization date. Overall survival (OS) was estimated according to the Kaplan-Meier method (Kaplan and Meier 1958). The prognostic importance of several variables with respect to TD was assessed using both univariate and multivariate methods. All p-values were two-sided. A p-value of less than 0.05 was considered to indicate significance. No correction of p-values for multiple analysis was performed.

As mentioned above, the study did not have the statistical power to detect small changes, as we were not interested in a small but statistically significant pain reduction in these patients with far advanced disease and considerable residual pain who were already on nonsteroidal anti-inflammatory drugs. Rather, we were searching for improvements which could be considered clinically relevant in this patient population.

Results

Patient Characteristics

Clinical characteristics of the study patients are listed in Table 4. Median age of the entire study population was 60.4 years: 58 years (range 37–82 years) in arm A and 62 years (range 39–88 years) in arm B. Twenty-nine patients had breast

Table 4. Patient characteristics SG 99/91

Characteristic	APD60 ($n=26$)	APD90 ($n=24$)
Gender, n (%)		
Male	5 (19)	4 (17)
Female	21 (81)	20 (83)
Histology, n (%)		
Breast	15 (58)	14 (58)
Myeloma	5 (19)	6 (25)
Urogenital	1 (4)	2 (8)
Prostate	1 (4)	0
Gastrointestinal	1 (4)	0
Cervix	1 (4)	0
Kidney	2 (8)	1 (4)
Unknown	0	1 (4)
Performance status, n (%)		
0–1	4 (15)	11 (46)
2	12 (46)	6 (25)
3	8 (31)	6 (25)
4	2 (8)	0
Unknown	0	1 (4)
Previous therapy, n (%)		
Hormone	4 (15)	6 (25)
Chemo	5 (19)	2 (8)
Hormone plus chemo	15 (58)	12 (50)
None	2 (8)	3 (13)
Unknown	0	1 (4)
Current therapy, n (%)		
Immuno plus hormone	4 (15)	3 (13)
Hormone plus chemo	5 (19)	3 (13)
None	9 (34)	11 (46)
Chemo	8 (31)	6 (25)
Unknown	0	1 (4)
Best response to current therapy, n (%)		
Partial response	1 (4)	1 (4)
No change	6 (23)	7 (29)
Progressive disease	18 (69)	15 (63)
Unknown	1 (4)	1 (4)
Age (years)		
Median	58	62
Range	37–82	39–89

Table 5. Patient characteristics SG 99/91

Characteristic	APD60 ($n=26$)	APD90 ($n=24$)
Physician-rated PSC, n (%)		
Mild	5 (19)	4 (17)
Moderate	6 (23)	12 (50)
Severe	9 (35)	5 (21)
Intractable	6 (23)	2 (8)
Unknown	0	1 (4)
Use of analgesics		
None	0	2 (8)
Paracetamol	1 (4)	2 (8)
NSAIDs	6 (23)	4 (17)
Opioids	4 (15)	7 (29)
Opiates	15 (58)	8 (33)
Unknown	0	1 (4)

cancer, 11 had myeloma and ten had other types of tumors. All patients received regular analgesic medication, modified WHO score >2. The mean analgesic score was 3.1 (range 2–4), the mean pain score was 2.4 (range 1–4), and the mean performance status was 2.1 (range 1–4). Details of physician-rated scores and LASA scales of the study patients are listed in Tables 5 and 6. Baseline laboratory values were similar in the two treatment arms, with the exception of AP (median 363 units/l in the 60-mg group versus 225 units/l in the 90-mg group; $p=0.03$) and osteocalcin (median 4.1 µg/l versus 4.5 µg/l, respectively; $p=0.10$). The institutional normal range for these parameters are 50–330 units/l and 2–12 µg/l, respectively. The baseline patients' characteristics together with LASA values were slightly imbalanced in favor of the 90-mg group. These patients had also a slightly better PS, lower PSC and PF, and used fewer analgesics with borderline significance (Tables 5, 6).

Properties of LASA Scales and PSC

At baseline, the LASA scales for PIN and PF were very significantly correlated ($r=0.51$, $p=0.0004$). As expected, WB was negatively correlated with PIN and PF ($r=0.22$, $p=0.16$ and $r=0.33$, $p=0.03$, respectively).

In addition, there was a significant linear trend between the patient-rated PIN and the categories of physician-rated PSC ($p=0.001$) at baseline. The trend was present at further time points.

Efficacy (LASA)

The overall mean values for LASA scales during treatment were always better for pamidronate 90 (borderline significance). However, this summary did not consider the rate of change in the two treatment arms.

Table 6. Patient characteristics SG 99/91

Characteristic	APD60 (n)	APD90 (n)
Total number of patients	26	24
Patient-rated PIN		
Median	61 (23)	58 (23)
Range	17–100	2–90
Patient-rated PF		
Median	79 (24)	63 (21)
Range	9–100	14–100
Patient-rated WB		
Median	34 (22)	38 (21)
Range	0–73	0–87
Osteocalcin (units/l)		
Median	4.1 (23)	5 (21)
Range	0.4–9.8	1.6–24.8
AP (units/l)		
Median	363 (23)	225 (21)
Range	101–4810	49–1134
Serum Ca (mmol/l)		
Median	2.45 (26)	2.4 (23)
Range	2.1–3	2–3.4
Urinary Ca/Crea		
Median	0.43 (24)	0.38 (20)
Range	0–2.1	0.04–1.3

Overall, the changes or improvements in LASA scales from entry were significantly different from zero: PIN ($p=0.0006$), PF ($p=0.0009$), WB ($p=0.001$). However, these changes in LASA scales were similar in both arms (slightly better for pamidronate 90). No significant difference was present for PIN, PF, and WB. A borderline difference was observed for PIM (median: 34 vs. 48 in the 60 vs. 90 group, $p=0.18$). Details of overall improvement can be seen in Table 7.

The changes or improvements in LASA scales form entry were compared in groups defined by selected patient characteristics (gender, breast tumors vs. others, current antitumor therapy Y/N, baseline performance status 0–1 vs. >1).

Overall, WB improvement was greater in men (median: 19 vs. 9, $p=0.14$), and in other tumors compared with breast tumors (median: 24 vs. 7, $p=0.03$). As expected, PIN reduction was larger in patients receiving antitumor therapy. However, this difference did not reach statistical significance (median –22 vs. –5, $p=0.16$).

PIN reduction was greater also in patients with worse performance status (median: –22 vs. –2, $p=0.04$). As expected, these patients already had greater pain intensity at baseline. Like PIN, PF reduction was greater in patients with worse performance status (median: –23 vs. –14, $p=0.08$).

Table 7. Efficacy (overall improvement): LASA and LAB SG 99/91

Parameter	APD60 (n = 26)	APD90 (n = 24)
Patient-rated PIN		
Median	−11 (18)	−22 (21)
Range	−65 to +19	−71 to +39
Patient-rated PF		
Median	−15 (19)	−23 (19)
Range	−67 to +50	−87 to +34
Patient-rated WB		
Median	12 (17)	10 (19)
Range	−23 to +40	−13 to +78
Osteocalcin		
Median	−0.90 (15)	−0.64 (17)
Range	−4.9 to +3.7	−2.3 to +3.4
AP		
Median	−8.7 (15)	3.3 (17)
Range	−122 to +1432	−220 to +1218
Serum Ca		
Median	−0.16 (22)	−0.13 (21)
Range	−0.8 to +0.10	−0.9 to +0.6
Urinary Ca/Crea		
Median	−0.14 (20)	−0.11 (18)
Range	−1.8 to +0.2	−1.2 to +2.6

It is well known that cancer patients with pain do not use LASA scales in a linear way. It seems that LASA scales for pain intensity do not measure pain intensity alone, but also other factors such as pain expectation and relation to analgesic therapy used or expected to be used. Factors other than pain intensity may influence self-assessment of cancer patients when they use this instrument. Patients frequently indicate a value different from zero using a LASA pain intensity instrument, even when the same patients say that they are actually free of pain. In this patient population with advanced cancer and pain there seems to be a lower limit of around 0.20–0.25 which acts as a threshold level. These factors have to be taken into consideration when conclusions are drawn from these results. Furthermore, it should be kept in mind that the LASA changes are strongly dependend on baseline values.

Multiple regression was used to assess treatment effect after adjustment for baseline scores and other covariates. After adjustment for gender, breast tumors vs. others, current antitumor therapy yes/no, baseline performance status 0–1 vs. >1, the randomized treatment regimen had a borderline association with reduction in PF (coeff: -14.1, $p = 0.09$), reduction of PIN (coeff: -10.9, $p = 0.08$), and reduction of PIM (coeff: 10.6, $p = 0.08$). With the exception of PIM (for which no baseline score was available), all LASA scale changes were strongly dependent on baseline scores.

The median percent change in PF after one infusion was –25% (–24% in pamidronate 60 and –25.6% in pamidronate 90). The median percent change in PF after one infusion was –10% (–10% in pamidronate 60 and –11% in pamidronate 90). With both PIN and PF, reduction means improvement of pain. The median percent increase in WB after one infusion was 18% (41% in pamidronate 60 and 3% in pamidronate 90). The median percent change in PIN after three infusions was –47% (–26% in pamidronate 60 and –54% in pamidronate 90). The median percent change in PF after three infusions was –39% (–9% in pamidronate 60 and –50% in pamidronate 90). The median percent increase in WB was 36% (36% in pamidronate 60 and 41% in pamidronate 90). Fewer patients in pamidronate 60 were in the study at the third infusion. See also treatment duration analysis. No comparative analysis was performed after the sixth infusion because of small patient numbers.

Efficacy (PS, PSC, and Use of Analgesics)

Performance Status. the poorest or "maximal" PS category 3 and 4 during treatment was observed in 7/22 (32%) vs. 11/22 (50%) patients in pamidronate 90 vs. pamidronate 60 ($p = 0.36$). Compared with baseline, an increase in PS (i.e., worsening of PS) was observed in 8/21 (38%) patients in pamidronate 90 vs. 9/22 (41%) patients in pamidronate 60 ($p = 0.98$). A decrease in PS (i.e., improving PS) was observed in 2/21 (10%) patients in pamidronate 90 vs. 2/22 (10%) patients in pamidronate 60.

Pain Score. The "maximal" PSC category 3 and 4 during treatment was observed in 6/22 (27%) patients in pamidronate 90 vs. 10/23 (43%) in pamidronate 60 ($p = 0.35$). Compared with baseline, an increase in PSC (i.e., worsening of PSC) was observed in 5/21 (24%) patients in pamidronate 90 vs. 8/23 (35%) in pamidronate 60 ($p = 0.35$). A decrease in PSC (i.e., improving PSC) was observed in 5/21 (24%) patients in pamidronate 90 vs. 6/23 (26%) in pamidronate 60.

Analgesic Use. Analgesics were reduced after the first administration of pamidronate in 8/24 (33%) patients in pamidronate 90 vs. 6/26 (23%) in pamidronate 60 ($p = 0.53$). The category of analgesic was "reduced" in 3/21 (14%) and 3/22 (14%) patients in pamidronate 90 and pamidronate 60, respectively, and "increased" in 2/21 (10%) and 6/22 (27%) patients in pamidronate 90 and in pamidronate 60, respectively ($p = 0.24$ for "increase" Y/N). The remaining patients continued to use the same category of analgesics during pamidronate treatment.

Efficacy (Laboratory Values)

Overall mean values for LAB parameters during treatment were always better for pamidronate 90 (borderline significance). The overall mean value for AP was significantly lower for pamidronate 90: median 199 units/l vs. 362 units/l ($p=0.02$). The overall mean value for OST was significantly higher for pamidronate 90: median 4.9 µg/l vs. 3.7 µg/l ($p<0.05$).

Overall, the changes or improvements in LAB values from entry differed highly significantly from zero for SCa ($p=0.0001$) and UCa/Cr ($p=0.0009$). The changes or improvements in LAB values from entry were similar for both arms (slightly better for pamidronate 90). No significant difference between the two arms was present for AP, OST, SCA, and UCa/Cr. Details of overall changes can be seen in Table 7.

After one infusion the median percent change of AP was 0.05%. The median percent change in OST was –14% (–20% in pamidronate 60 and –8% in pamidronate 90). The median percent change in SCa was –4% (in both arms). The median percent decrease in UCa/Cr was –62% (–62% in pamidronate 60 and –64% in pamidronate 90). Details of efficacy after one infusion (analyzed as percent improvement) are summarized in Table 8. After three infusions the median percent change in AP was –12% (–9% in pamidronate 60 and –15% in pamidronate 90). The median percent decrease in SCa was

Table 8. Efficacy (percent improvement after one infusion): LASA and LAB SG 99/91

Parameter	APD60 (n = 26)	APD90 (n = 24)
Patient-rated PIN		
Median	–0.24 (17)	–0.26 (19)
Range	–0.88 to +0.65	–1 to 30.5
Patient-rated PF		
Median	–0.10 (18)	–0.11 (18)
Range	–0.83 to +1.1	–0.98 to +0.52
Patient-rated WB		
Median	0.41 (14)	0.03 (15)
Range	–0.41 to +7	–0.4 to +1.9
Osteocalcin (units/l)		
Median	–0.20 (14)	–0.08 (16)
Range	–0.78 to +1.7	–0.66 to +2.25
AP (units/l)		
Median	–0.01 (15)	0.02 (17)
Range	–0.3 to +1.24	–0.28 to +1.60
Serum Ca (mmol/l)		
Median	–0.04 (20)	–0.04 (19)
Range	–0.29 to +0.09	–0.35 to +0.21
Urinary Ca/Crea		
Median	–0.62 (15)	–0.64 (16)
Range	–0.91 to +1.09	–0.90 to +6.63

Table 9. Efficacy (percent improvement after three infusions): LASA and LAB SG 99/91

Parameter	APD60 (n = 26)	APD90 (n = 24)
Patient-rated PIN		
Median	−0.26 (10)	−0.54 (17)
Range	−0.96 to +0.85	−1 to +15.5
Patient-rated PF		
Median	−0.09 (10)	−0.50 (14)
Range	−0.86 to +1.09	−1 to +1.03
Patient-rated WB		
Median	0.36 (9)	0.41 (14)
Range	−0.79 to +2.2	−0.57 to +1.8
Osteocalcin (units/l)		
Median	−0.09 (6)	−0.15 (12)
Range	−0.43 to +1.3	−1 to +2.06
AP (units/l)		
Median	−0.07 (6)	−0.14 (12)
Range	−0.43 to +0.29	−0.36 to +1.21
Serum Ca (mmol/l)		
Median	−0.06 (12)	−0.04 (15)
Range	−0.23 to +0.04	−0.15 to +0.09
Urinary Ca/Crea		
Median	−0.02 (13)	−0.43 (16)
Range	−0.96 to +0.38	−1 to +0.02

−4% (−6% in pamidronate 60 and −4% in pamidronate 90). The median percent decrease in UCa/Cr was −33% (−22% in pamidronate 60 and −43% in pamidronate 90). As for the LASA, fewer patients in pamidronate 60 were on study at the third cycle. See also treatment duration analysis. Details of efficacy after three infusions (analyzed as percent improvement) are summarized in Table 9. No formal analysis was performed after six infusions because of the low number of patients.

Treatment Duration

All patients were off treatment at the time of evaluation. The median treatment duration was longer in the pamidronate 90 group: 101 vs. 44 days in the pamidronate 60 group ($p = 0.05$). The reason for stopping treatment was generally death (seven in each arm), but also treatment not necessary = no pain (5/26 pamidronate 60 vs. 9/24 pamidronate 90) and patient dissatisfaction (13/26 pamidronate 60 vs. 3/24 pamidronate 90), which occurred more frequently in the pamidronate 60 arm: $p = 0.006$. Other causes were: protocol violation (one pamidronate 90), lost to follow-up (one pamidronate 90), patient and physician decision (one in each arm). OS is similar in the two treatment arms (data not shown).

Toxicity and Side Effects

Overall tolerance was excellent. In the pamidronate-60 arm, one case of fever after the first and after the second infusion and one case of increased bone pain after the fifth infusion were observed. In the pamidronate-90 arm, one patient had fever and phlebitis, seen during several visits, and another patient had an episode of phlebitis after the first and the fifth infusion.

Multivariate Analysis

In an attempt to adjust for baseline values and other covariates such as gender, histological diagnosis, concomitant anticancer therapy, and baseline performance status, multiple regression analysis was performed to gain a better estimate of treatment effect on the study population. Again, a trend was seen in favor of the treatment regimen using 90 mg pamidronate, with regard to a reduction in pain intensity, pain frequency, and pain improvement. The respective p-values were 0.08, 0.09, and 0.08. Regarding the primary end point of the study, the following observations can be made: The mean reduction in pain intensity was 26% in the 60-mg group and 54% in the 90-mg group. A similar result was seen in pain frequency after three infusions, 9% vs. 50%. Accordingly, the median increase in well-being was 36% with 60 mg and 41% with 90 mg pamidronate. Most interesting was the finding that patients (and physicians) continued treatment for an average of 2.1 infusions with the lower dose but for an average of 4.8 infusions with the higher dose. At least three infusions were intended, but treatment could be stopped early based on the patient's and the physician's decision, influenced mainly by the achievement of complete pain relief or the patient's dissatisfaction due to low efficacy. An analysis of reasons for stopping treatment showed a favorable outcome for patients treated with a higher dose: nine of 24 patients (38%) treated with the high dose but only five of 26 (19%) treated with the lower dose stopped treatment because they achieved complete pain relief. On the other hand, only three of 24 patients treated with the higher dose regimen (13%) but 13 of 26 patients (50%) treated with the lower dose regimen reported dissatisfaction with the treatment and discontinued it. The difference between the treatment groups was highly significant ($p=0.006$). The effectiveness of pamidronate in reducing bone resorption was underlined by the highly significant LAB values. The median decrease in urinary calcium creatinine ratio (UCa/CR) was in excess of 60% with both treatments ($p=0.0009$), with a trend to increase with time despite progression of the disease in the majority of the patients. After the third infusion, the median reduction in UCa/CR was 22% with 60 mg and 43% with 90 mg pamidronate. There was also a statistically significant decrease in the median serum calcium values of 4% compared with baseline ($p=0.0001$). For treatment effects over time see also Figs. 8–13. Asterix indicates earliest visit with significant difference of study parameter compared to baseline value. SEM indicates standard error of the mean.

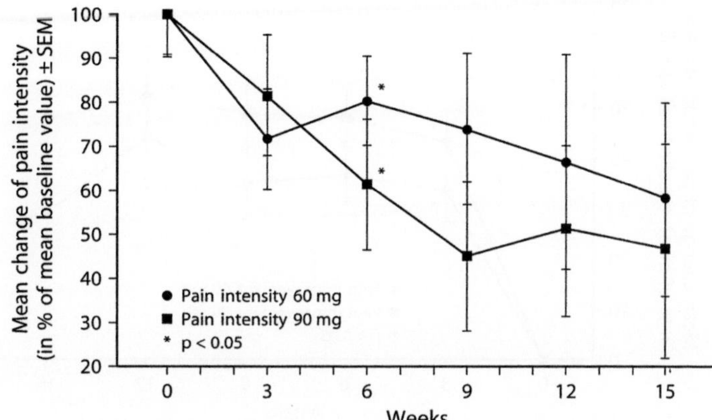

Fig. 8. Effects of pamidronate treatment on pain intensity in SG 99/91 protocol

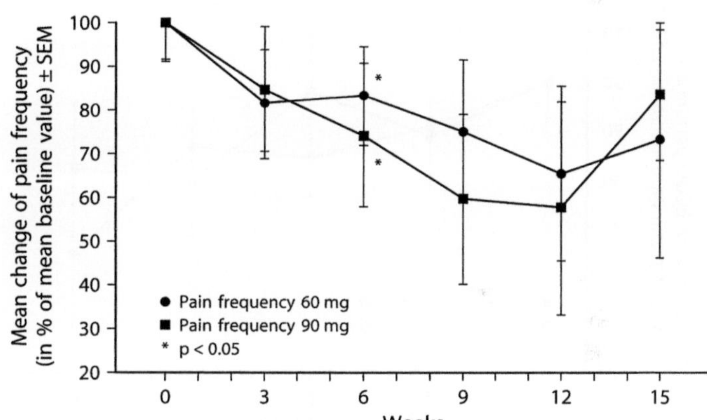

Fig. 9. Effects of pamidronate treatment on pain frequency in SG 99/91 protocol

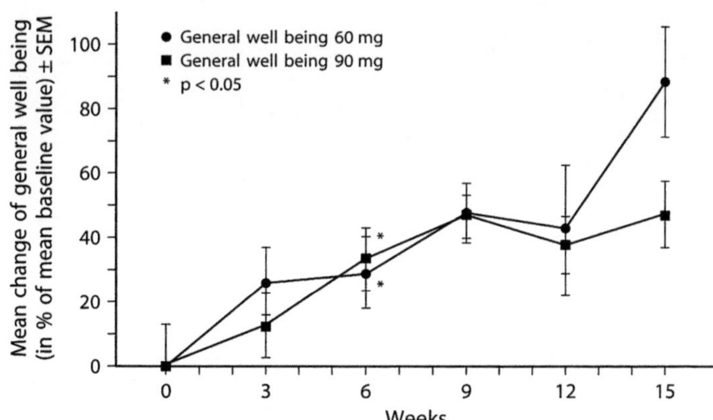

Fig. 10. Effects of pamidronate treatment on general well-being in SG 99/91 protocol

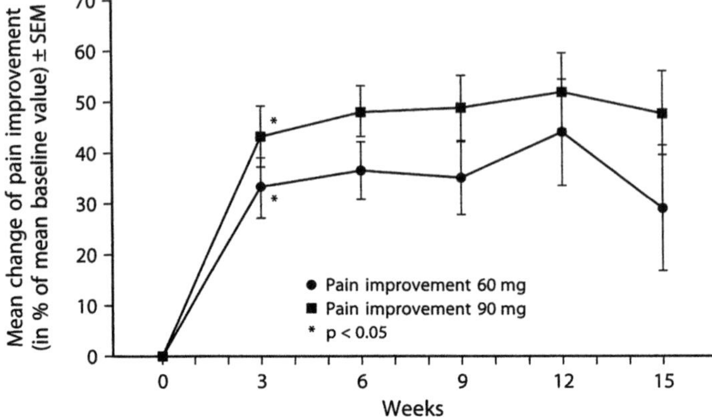

Fig. 11. Effects of pamidronate treatment on pain improvement in SG 99/91 protocol

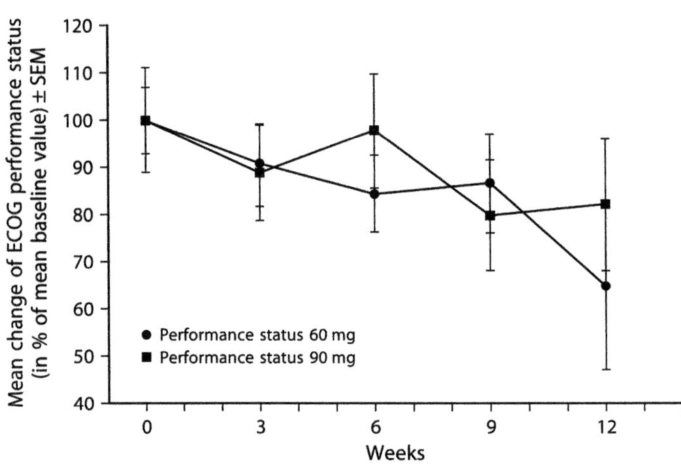

Fig. 12. Effects of pamidronate treatment on ECOG performance status in SG 99/91 protocol

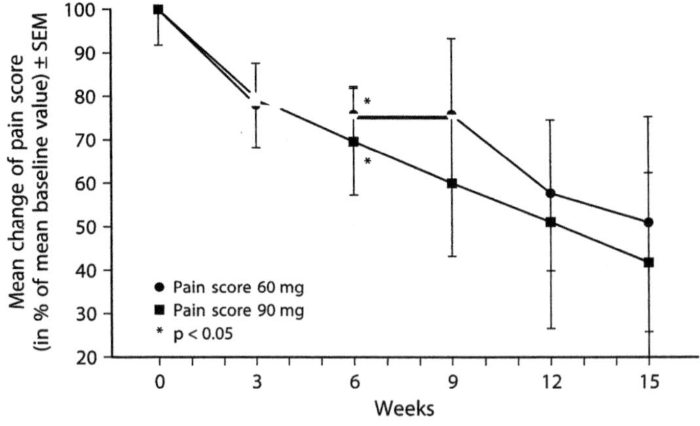

Fig. 13. Effects of pamidronate treatment on pain score in SG 99/91 protocol

Conclusion

The results of our prospective randomized study show a significant improvement in pain and other relevant parameters of palliation using both 60 and 90 mg of pamidronate. Subjective parameters assessed by patients using LASA correlated well with physician assessments and with laboratory parameters monitoring bone resorption. There was a trend towards better palliation for the treatment regimen with a higher dose intensity. Several parameters such as duration of treatment and patient dissatisfaction showed a statistically significant difference in favor of the 90 mg regimen. However, caution is indicated in the interpretation of the results, because treatment was not assigned and administered in double-blind fashion. The knowledge that they were being treated with the higher dose might well have influenced the patients' and/or the physicians' decision to continue treatment. In order to eliminate this possible source of error, a double-blind prospective randomized study would be more appropriate to investigate the effect of two different doses on partially subjective study parameters. (See study SG 110/93).

References

Bernhard J, Huerny C, Bacchi M, et al for the Swiss Group for Clinical Cancer Research (SAKK) (1996) Initial prognostic factors in small cell lung cancer patients predicting quality of life during chemotherapy. Br J Cancer 348:563–566

Cuzick J (1995) A Wilcoxon-type test for trend. Stat Med 4:87–90

Hopwood P, Stephens RJ, Machin D (1994) Approches to the analysis of quality of life data: experiences gained from the Medical Research Council lung cancer working party palliative chemotherapy trial. Qual Life Res 3:339–352

Kaplan EL, Meier P (1958) Nonparametric estimation from incomplete observations. Am Stat Assoc 53:457–481

Neter J, Wassermann W, Kutner MH (1985) Applied linear statistical models. Regression, analysis of variance and experimental designs. Irwin, Homewood, Ill., USA

Robertson AG, Reed NS, Ralston SH (1995) Effect of oral clodronate on metastatic bone pain: a double-blind, placebo-controlled study. J Clin Oncol 13:2427–2430

Pamidronate Versus Controls in Patients with Metastatic Breast Cancer and Bone Metastases

Pamidronate for Inhibition of Bone Progression in Patients with Advanced Breast Cancer: A Randomized, Multicenter Phase-III Trial

Concomitant with the aforementioned study, SG 99/91, our institution participated in a prospective randomized trial, along with others in the Aredia Multinational Cooperative Group, to evaluate the ability of pamidronate given with chemotherapy to delay the progression of bone disease in patients with breast cancer and skeletal metastases. This question was examined in a patient population which was much less advanced in their disease and had had no prior chemotherapy for advanced disease; half of the patients had received no prior systemic antineoplastic treatment for advanced disease at all, whereas the other half had had prior endocrine therapy for metastasic disease. Median time since diagnosis of bone metastases was only 2–3 months. Details of the study have been reported elsewhere (Conte et al. 1994).

Patients and Methods

A total of 295 patients were entered in the study, of whom 152 were randomized to chemotherapy alone and 143 to chemotherapy plus pamidronate 45 mg intravenously every 3 weeks. The chemotherapy regimen for first-line treatment was standardized in each participating institution and was given until undue toxicity or progressive disease was observed, or for maximum of 6–12 cycles as recommended by the treating physician. Pamidronate was given until toxicity or progressive bone disease was observed. Patients were examined every 3 weeks. Skeletal X-rays were repeated every 3 months and bone scans every 6 months (earlier in cases with increased bone pain and/or bone-related complications). The primary end point of the study was time to bone progression and reduction in bone pain. X-rays and bone scans were reviewed *extra muros* under blinded conditions. Bone pain was evaluated on a six-point self-assessment scale, and categories of patients showing minor improvement (by one point over two consecutive reports or by two points in one report) or marked improvement (defined as improvement by two points over at least two consecutive reports) were assigned. Secondary end points included time to progressive disease in bone according to the individual investigator, overall incidence of bone-related complications (orthopedic surgery, pathological fractures, need for radiotherapy, episodes of hypercalcemia), sclerotic responses of lytic lesions, response of extraskeletal metastases, and overall survival. Bone progression curves and survival curves were analyzed according to the Kaplan-Meier method and compared using the t-test; categories of pain changes were compared using the chi-square test.

Results

Extramural reviews of all imaging studies were undertaken for 240/283 evaluable patients (79% of the entire study population). Median time to tumor progression in bone was 249 days in the pamidronate-treated group and 168 days in the control group ($p = 0.02$; see Fig. 14. According to the individual investigators, median time to progressive bone disease was 333 days and 209 days, respectively, for the two groups ($p = 0.02$).

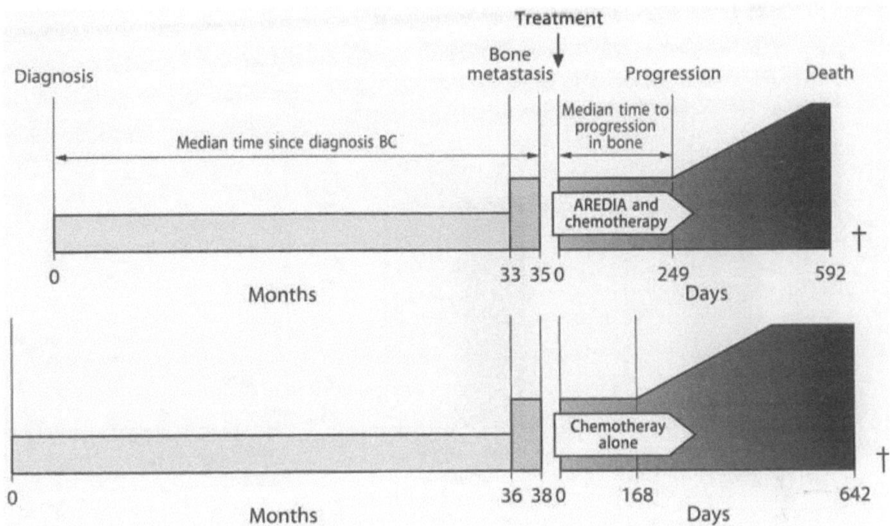

Fig. 14. Pamidronate used in the indication of osteolytic bone metastases. *BC* breast cancer

Overall, 227 patients (84%) had bone pain at the time of randomization. During the trial, 61% of patients in the pamidronate group and 51% of the patients in the control group reported no pain. Minor pain improvement was reported in 65% of the patients receiving pamidronate and in 60% of those in the control arm. Marked pain improvement was noted in 44% of the patients treated with pamidronate and in 30% of those treated with chemotherapy only ($p = 0.025$).

Bone-related complications occurred in 65/116 patients in the pamidronate arm and in 68/108 patients in the control arm. Some patients developed more than one complication. The overall numbers of complications were 135 and 169 in the pamidronate and control arms, respectively. Median time for the first bone-associated complication was 533 days for patients receiving pamidronate and 490 days for controls. Median time to first radiotherapy was 697 days for pamidronate and 571 days for controls (Fig. 15). All these differences were not statistically significant. Sclerotic response of lytic lesions was documented in 53% of the patients treated with pamidronate and in 44% of controls. The overall response rate of extraskeletal disease was similar in the two groups, i.e., 34% versus 31%, as was median survival: 592 versus 642 days for the pamidronate group and the control group, respectively (Fig. 14). The overall effectiveness of Aredia and chemotherapy versus chemotherapy alone is summarized in Fig. 16.

Discussion

The results of this multicenter study showed clearly that intravenous pamidronate given at a dose of 45 mg every 3 weeks with chemotherapy signifi-

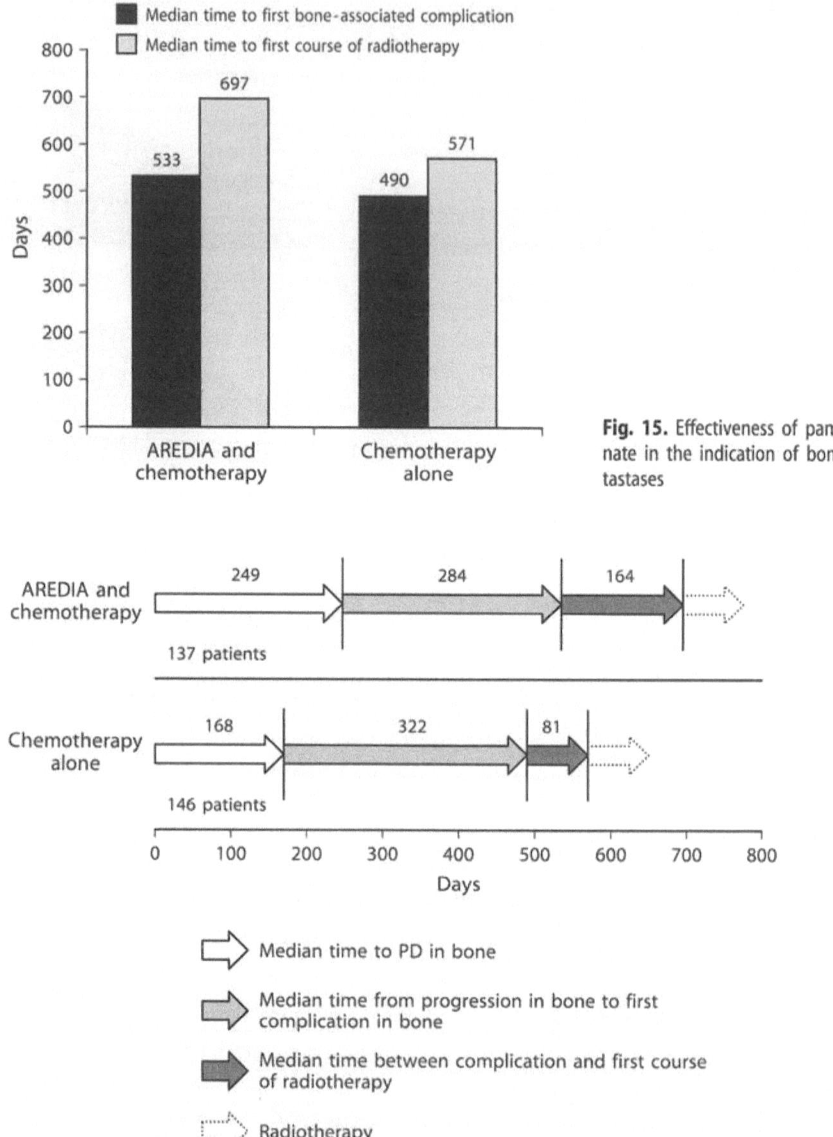

Fig. 15. Effectiveness of pamidronate in the indication of bone metastases

Fig. 16. Overall effectiveness of pamidronate plus chemotherapy versus chemotherapy alone in the indication of bone metastases

cantly delays progression of bone metastases in comparison to the same chemotherapy alone in patients with advanced breast cancer. The interpretation of serial X-rays and of bone scans by the treating physician may be biased because of the nonblinded fashion of the study. While it is true that a double-blind, placebo-controlled trial would have been preferable, the administration of intravenous placebo every 3 weeks for an indefinite period was considered unacceptable by many physicians. In an attempt to correct for this methodological weakness, an external review under strictly blinded conditions was performed by one radiologist and one oncologist per country. This blinded external review also showed a statistically significant prolongation of the median time of bone progression using pamidronate. The conclusions of the review are in line with the data reported by the individual investigators. Longer follow-up and the greater number of patients evaluated by the individual investigators may account for the extended median times of progression seen by the latter compared with the reviewed data. The treatment effect of pamidronate did not translate into a significant reduction of bone-related complications, however, although there was a clear trend to fewer complications in the pamidronate group. The results of most parameters investigated were in favor of pamidronate added to chemotherapy. There are several possible explanations for the lack of a significant reduction in bone-related complications in this study. The overall incidence of such complications is low, as expected. Treatment was given in a rather early stage of the disease – when first-line chemotherapy was started. Pathological fractures occurred in only 18% of all patients, and orthopedic surgery was needed in only a small minority of patients. Hypercalcemic episodes were rare and seen in only 7% of the patients. The high degree of effectiveness of chemotherapy given as first-line treatment in this group of patients with advanced breast cancer most probably also contributed to the low incidence of complications in the treatment group. Furthermore, the relatively short period of observation with a median follow-up of less than 18 months and the relatively low proportion of patients who had shown bone progression at the time of analysis – 40% – also contributed to the low number of complications. These results clearly lead us to question at which point in time during the course of the disease should pamidronate treatment be started? Criteria for adequate selection of the patient population which would benefit most are needed. The dose of 45 mg pamidronate given every 3 weeks could also be challenged: 15 mg pamidronate every 3 weeks might be appropriate for inhibition of bone progression in a patient population with less advanced disease than the one used in this study. On the other hand, several nonrandomized studies of patients with advanced disease showed best palliative effects using higher doses (Hacking et al. 1991; Morton et al. 1989). Our previously described dose-escalation study and the results of two dose-finding trials in patients with breast and prostate cancer generated by an American group also showed uniformly that higher doses and/or dose intensities gave superior results; e.g., in the latter study, performed in patients with breast cancer, a pamidronate regimen of 30 mg every 2 weeks did not produce significant effects regarding reduction of bone pain or biochemical parameters of bone resorption, while consistent reductions in these parameters were observed with regimens involving higher doses: 60 mg every 2 weeks and 90 mg every 4 weeks. A further regimen, albeit using 60 mg but given only every 4 weeks, produced intermediate results. All these studies lead to the conclusion that there is a clear relation between palliative effect and dose/ dose intensity administered, at least in the range of 30–60 mg pamidronate as a single dose and for dose intensities in the range of 12.5–20.5 mg pamidronate per week in breast cancer patients with advanced bone disease. However, optimal schedules – single doses, dose time intervals, start of treatment, and duration of treatment – for different patient populations require further investigation.

The dose-effect relationship might also exist in patients with breast cancer and less advanced bone disease. A smaller prospective randomized study from the United Kingdom showed that 30 mg pamidronate given intravenously every 3 weeks had no statistically significant effect in breast cancer patients undergoing hormone treatment with aminoglutethimide and hydrocortisone. Obviously, this patient population had even less advanced disease than the patients in the Aredia Multinational Cooperative Study reported above. Although there was a trend favoring pamidronate-treated patients in this British study, this difference did not reach statistical significance. Possible explanations are the small sample size reported (76 patients), the low number of events among these patients, or the fact that the chosen dose was too low for this patient population (Harris et al. 1991).

References

Conte PF, Gianessi PG, Latraile J, et al (1994) Delayed progression of bone metastases with pamidronate therapy in breast cancer patients: randomised multicenter phase III-trial. Ann Oncol 5:41–44

Hacking A, Gudegeon CA, McNorton MAC, et al (1991) Pamidronate (APD) as single infusion monotherapy in the treatment of bone metastasis from breast cancer. In: Bijvoet OLM, Lipton A (eds) Osteoclast inhibition in the management of malignancy related bone disorders. Hogrefe and Huber, Livingston, pp 45–53

Harris AL, Milward M, Tompkin K, et al (1991) Randomised trial of aminoglutethamide and hydrocortisone with and without disodium pamidronate in patients with advanced postmenopausal breast cancer and bone metastasis. In: Bijvoet OLM, Lipton A (eds) Osteoclast inhibition in the management of malignancy related bone disorders. Hogrefe and Huber, Livingston, pp 65–73

Morton A, Dodwell DJ, Howell A (1989) Disodium pamidronate infusion for bone metastasis: clinical trial in patients with breast carcinoma. In: Burckart P (ed) Disodium pamidronate in the treatment of malignancy related disorders. Huber, Toronto, pp 120–133

Aredia in the Indication of Osteolytic Bone Metastases of Breast Cancer: A Model for Evaluation of Cost-Benefit

A pharmacoeconomic model for estimating the impact of pamidronate on the evolution of bone metastases has also been applied to this study. The long-term pharmacoeconomic impact of pamidronate in the evolution of bone metastases was evaluated retrospectively in the previously conducted multicenter prospective randomized phase III study in patients with advanced breast cancer and bone metastases receiving first-line chemotherapy. Analysis concentrated on the quality of life with respect to the treatment, the observed complications of bone metastases, the time to progressive disease in bone, the time to first radiotherapy, and the performance status. Measures of quality of life were evaluated using the Rosser scale, relating degrees of disability to distress ratings in terms of quality-adjusted life years (QUALYs). The gain in QUALYs before progressive disease in bone plus the days to first complication, plus the gain in days to first radiotherapy amounted to a total of 21.4 QUALYs per 100 patients. Analysis of the economic impact was restricted to cost elements because the clinical trial did not include any prospectively specified pharmacoeconomic end points. We analyzed costs for treatment of bone metastases in ten consecutive patients with advanced malignancy and bone metastases referred to our unit in the Kantonsspital St. Gallen. The average cost was used to calculate the treatment costs of pamidronate and the costs that were avoided for radiotherapy and surgery. Only these direct costs have been included in the analysis. Additional costs caused by the application of non-cost covering tariffs in the hospital were not taken into account. Fees for outpatient treatment and operations were used according to the tariff of the Swiss Medical Association, and hospital costs were determined using ALS Swiss Hospital Statistics.

Possible indirect benefits of pamidronate treatment, such as gain in pain-free days, improved quality of life, less diagnostic workup and fewer changes in antineoplastic therapy, postponement of bone progression, and possible benefits of avoided indirect costs due to fewer days in hospital and fewe repisodes of radiotherapy were not taken into account.

The total cost per treatment cycle using this model amounted to 303.85 SFr. The average treatment cost per patient amounted to 3600 SFr (Table 10). The

Table 10. Treatment costs with Aredia, administered at 3-week intervals as a 1-h infusion of 45 mg

Cost factors	Sfr	Ecu[a]
Medication		
Aredia 45 mg (3 units)	256.50	157.40
Saline (0.9%) 500 ml	5.60	3.45
Infusion set	1.35	0.83
Nursing time 30 min	24.75	15.20
Doctor's visit: one visit every 9 weeks		
Fee (tariff: Swiss Med. Assoc.)	15.65	9.60
	303.85	184.48
Control examination		
Serum creatinine (Sfr 22.00)×0.1	2.20	
Serum calcium (Sfr 22.00)×0.1	2.20	
	4.40	2.70
Total costs per cycle	303.85	184.48
Average treatment costs per patient (35.6 weeks = 11.85 cycles)	3600	2209

[a] 1 Ecu = Sfr 1.63 (July 1994).

reduced radiotherapy cost per treatment course and the reduced cost for surgery per case were estimated to be 2000 SFr and 14,000 SFr, respectively (Table 11). Tables 12 and 13 give an overview of types of potential benefits and avoided costs associated with pamidronate treatment.

The cost-benefit comparison showed that costs in the pamidronate arm were 3600 SFr for 100% of the patients treated ($n = 137$). The average costs in the pamidronate arm were 960 SFr for radiotherapy, required by 48% of the patients, and 406 SFr for surgery, required by 2.9% of the patients. In the control arm ($n = 146$) the costs for pamidronate treatment were obviously zero, whereas costs for radiotherapy were 1260 SFr, required by 63% of the patients, and 770 SFr for surgery, required by 5.5% of the patients (Table 14). The total cost per patient treated would therefore amount to 4072 SFr in the pamidronate arm

Table 11. Costs of complications of bone metastases

	Sfr	Ecu[a]
Radiotherapy, one series	2000,–[b]	1227,–
Surgery for long-bone fracture[c]		
Humerus (ALS 15.8 d)	12000,–	7362,–
Femur (ALS 23.7 d)	16000,–	9816,–

[a] 1 Ecu =: Sfr 1.63 (July 1994).
[b] Low estimate.
[c] Operation cost (Tariff Swiss Med. Assoc.); hospitalization cost (ALS Swiss hospital statistics).

Table 12. Benefits of treatment with Aredia

Benefit	Type of gain
Gain in pain-free days	Intangible
Improved quality of life	Intangible
Less change in chemotherapy	Monetary: direct and indirect costs
Postponement of progression	Intangible and monetary: indirect costs
Fewer operations due to long-bone fractures	Monetary: direct costs
Fewer days in hospital	Monetary: direct and indirect costs
Fewer episodes of radiotherapy	Monetary: direct and indirect costs

Table 13. Costs avoided through treatment with Aredia

	Monetary value	
	Sfr	Ecu[a]
1. Postponement of progression	Intangible	
2. Improved quality of life	Intangible	
3. Reduced radiotherapy requirement (per session)	2000	1227
4. Reduced requirement for surgery (average)	14000	8589

[a] 1 Ecu = Sfr 1.63 (July 1994).

Table 14. Cost-benefit comparison of treatment with Aredia (in SFr; percent of cases treated)

	Medication	Episodes of radiotherapy	Episodes of surgery
Aredia, 137 = 100%	3600 (100%)	960 (48%)	406 (2.9%)
Control, 146 = 100%	(0%)	1260 (63%)	770 (5.5%)

and 841 SFr in the control arm. The cost for the 0.21 QUALYS gained by an average patient treated with pamidronate are 3231 SFr. As mentioned before, these costs do not take the avoided indirect costs into consideration and have to be compared with costs of other health interventions.

Other groups also investigated the cost-benefit aspects of clodronate and pamidronate therapy to reduce common complicatons of breast cancer, using models which take prices and costs (as of November 1993) of the health-care system in the United Kingdom into account. The analysis showed that the cost of pamidronate treatment (60 mg given intravenously every month) compared with the financial savings due to reduced costs for the treatment of complications approximately break even, whereas the cost of clodronate treatment (1600 mg orally per day) was over four times higher than the cost of treating the complications as they arise. These limited cost-benefit data indicate that pamidronate treatment "breaks even," in that the costs of preventing complications are equal to the cost of treating bone-associated complications of patients with advanced breast cancer.

More favorable clinical and pharmacoeconomic results for clodronate were found in a Finnish study, in which 350 myeloma patients received standard melphalan-prednisolone chemotherapy and were randomized to 2400 mg oral clodronate per day or placebo for a total of 2 years. The proportion of patients with bone progression was twice as high in the placebo group as in the clodronate group (24% versus 12%; $p = 0.026$). Subgroup analysis showed that all patients, irrespective of age, sex, stage, presence of lytic lesions, or vertebral fractures, had a positive effect from clodronate treatment. The only subgroup that showed no benefit were patients who did not respond to cytotoxic treatment. Length of hospital stay was shorter and hospital costs were lower by 12% in the clodronate group (difference not significant), but total costs (including clodronate treatment and hospital costs) were 18% lower in the placebo group (not significant). Other factors and indirect costs are included in this analysis, which was based on the stucture of the Finnish health-care system. It was concluded that the additional costs of clodronate treatment are moderate when the improved quality of life is taken into account (Laakso et al. 1994).

References

Laakso A, Lahtinen R, Virkkunen P, Elomaa I, for the Finnish Leukaemia Group (1994) Subgroup and cost-benefit analysis of the Finnish multicentre trial of clodronate in multiple myeloma. Br J Haematol 8:725–729

Prospective, Randomized, Double-blind, Dose-finding Study in Patients with Malignant Osteolytic Bone Metastases and Pain: 60 mg vs. 90 mg Pamidronate (SG 110/93)

Introduction

Pamidronate and other bisphosphonates are effective in the treatment of pain due to osteolytic bone metastases and can be given safely to patients with normal kidney function in an outpatient setting. When the administration guidelines were adhered to, no relevant side effects were observed except for mild phlebitis and an acute-phase reaction due to cytokine release in a small minority of patients. Rarely, transient increased bone pain is reported with bisphosphonate infusions. Our previously conducted study, which tested pamidronate 60 mg vs. 90 mg intravenously every 3 weeks, showed that final interpretation of the data would be possible only if the drug could be administered in a double-blind fashion. The analysis of baseline data of the previous randomized study (SG 99/91) showed an imbalance of the main baseline values for pain intensity on the LASA scale between the treatment groups. We therefore stratified not only according to diagnosis, but also according to pain intensity on the LASA scale at baseline.

We used virtually the same inclusion and exclusion criteria as in the previously conducted non-double-blind study but modified the eligibility criteria regarding analgesic requirements prior to randomization. Patients were eligible only if they had been treated with full-dose nonsteroidal anti-inflammatory drugs (corresponding to our modified WHO analgesics score 2): e.g., 200 mg diclofenac per day, 1800–2400 mg ibuprofen per day, or 40 mg piroxicam per day. The patients also had to be on regular analgesics.

Furthermore, additional secondary study end points were added. New methods for determining bone degradation and bone formation products in the serum and in the urine were introduced, and bone mineral density measurements were planned at baseline, after three infusions, and after six infusions or at the time when patients went off the study.

Aim of the Study

The trial investigated the effect on pain and other parameters which are important for quality of life. The patients estimated the treatment effects using LASA scales for pain intensity, pain frequency, pain improvement, and general well-being by completing a patient questionnaire, whereas the physicians rated pain score, performance status, and analgesic score. Biochemical analysis of parameters for bone resorption and formation, remineralization of osteolysis on X-rays, and total body bone densitometry also had to be used to estimate treatment effects.

Study Design

The trial was conducted as a prospective, randomized, parallel double-blind study. Randomization was done in blocks of five patients to ensure balanced patient characteristics between the treatment arms. Stratification factors included diagnosis (breast cancer versus myeloma versus other malignancy) and pain intensity on LASA scale at baseline (<50 mm vs. >50 mm). Randomization was done by the research nurse of the Department of Internal Medicine C, Kantonsspital St. Gallen, after she had performed an eligibility check and been informed about the patient's identification, the name of the physician in charge, the diagnosis, and the LASA scale value for pain intensity at baseline. The infusions were also prepared by the research nurse and then administered by the regular nursing staff on the wards or in the outpatient department. At no time during the study was the research nurse involved in the acquisition of data, documentation of the study – except for the above-mentioned eligibility check and randomization procedures – or analysis of the study. The study was approved by the local ethical review board.

Inclusion criteria included histologically or cytologically proven malignancy, osteolytic bone disease, WHO pain score ≥ 2 while taking regular analgesics, modified WHO analgesic score ≥ 2 at full daily doses, adequate organ functions with serum creatinine <350 µmol/l, and written informed consent.

Exclusion criteria were terminal malignant disease, pregnancy or lactation, age <20 years, exposure to bisphosphonates, and recently begun hormone treatment, both within 4 weeks prior to study entry. Concomitant use of other bisphosphonates, concomitant medication with corticosteroids except for pulse dose therapy given <7 days in conjunction with chemotherapy, and concomitant radiotherapy to the only or all pain localizations (pain assessment outside of the radiated area must be possible) were not allowed. Failure to fulfill one inclusion criterion excluded a patient from the study.

Treatment

The patient received 60 mg or 90 mg pamidronate in at least 250 ml 0.9% NaCl intravenously over 2 h, repeated every 3 weeks. When new safety data on the infusion rate emerged during the study, the minimal infusion time required was shortened to 90 min. Treatment was planned to be continued until the patient and/or the physician decided that continuation was not in the patient's best interests. However, at least three infusions were planned, and treatment was usually stopped after six infusions.

Statistical Considerations

The primary parameter for sample size calculation was pain intensity on the LASA scale. For the detection of a 50% difference in the LASA scale value between the two treatment arms after three infusions, nine evaluable patients per treatment arm were necessary, considering an α-error of 0.05 and a power of 0.8. A baseline value of 50 mm and a reduction of pain intensity to 40 mm (20%) in the treatment arm with the lower dose was assumed. Twelve evaluable patients per arm after three infusions would be necessary to detect the same difference with a power of 0.9. For this calculation a standard deviation of dose intensity of 1.5 was assumed. The above-mentioned considerations for analysis were made at the time of the protocol preparation, when preliminary results of the nonblinded study SG 99/91 were available. Mean pain intensity at study entry of the patients randomized to 60 mg ($n = 24$) was 57.65±24.79; this was reduced to 39.4±22.6 ($n = 20$) after one infusion and to 46.63±30.12 ($n = 8$) after three infusions. Patients in the 90-mg arm started with a mean pain intensity LASA value of 52.18±23.77 ($n = 22$); their pain intensity was reduced to 41.95±28.23 ($n = 19$) after one infusion and finally to a mean of 25.31±17.73 ($n = 13$) after three infusions. We were well aware that further considerations might be necessary whenever newer results of the ongoing study were available, especially should the differences between the treatment groups with longer follow-up become smaller. It was therefore decided to include at least 40 patients in the study. In 1995 it was decided to increase the sample size to at least 70 patients in order to be able to detect also a smaller difference between the treatment arms.

Patient Characteristics

Between November 1993 and February 1996, 70 patients were included and treated on the study. The majority of patients were female (56 of 70) and had breast cancer. Mean age was about 62 years, with a range of 38–82 years. Forty-nine patients received chemotherapy and five patients hormone therapy, whereas 16 patients received no antineoplastic therapy for their underlying malignancy. Only three patients achieved a partial remission; 26 patients had disease stabilization, and 41 patients had progression of their malignancy as the best response during the study period. Patients randomized to the 90-mg group had slightly less favorable baseline characteristics regarding pain intensity and pain score. They also used slightly more potent analgesics and had a slightly worse performance status. However, none of these differences in baseline characteristics were statistically significant. The mean number of infusions administered to the patients was similar in both groups: 5.1 and 5.2 (range 1–6), respectively. Futher details can be seen in Table 15.

Table 15. Patient characteristics at entry to study SG 110/93

Characteristic	Pamidronate 60 mg $n=35$ (%)	Pamidronate 90 mg $n=35$ (%)
Sex		
Male	8 (23%)	6 (17%)
Female	27 (77%)	29 (83%)
Mean age, years (range)	62 (38–82)	63 (38–80)
Diagnosis		
Breast cancer	21 (60%)	21 (60%)
Multiple myeloma	8 (23%)	8 (23%)
Other tumors[a]	6 (17%)	6 (17%)
Skeletal metastases as only site of disease	24 (69%)	18 (51%)
Concomitant antineoplastic therapy		
Chemotherapy	26 (74%)	23 (66%)
Hormonal treatment	2 (6%)	3 (8%)
No antineoplastic therapy	7 (20%)	9 (26%)
Best response during study		
Partial response	2 (6%)	1 (3%)
Stable disease	14 (40%)	12 (34%)
Progressive disease	19 (54%)	22 (63%)
Radiotherapy during study	4 (11%)	6 (17%)
Pain intensity, mean (±SEM)[b]	49.97 (±3.2)	54.71 (±3.6)
Pain score, mean (±SEM)	2.03 (±0.2)	2.17 (±0.2)
Analgesic score, mean (±SEM)	2.91 (±0.2)	3.23 (±0.2)
ECOG performance status, mean (±SEM)	1.51 (±0.2)	1.69 (±0.2)

[a] One head and neck tumor, three prostate cancers, one pancreatic cancer, one cancer of unknown origin in the 60-mg group; one carcinoma of the cervix, one non-cell lung cancer, two prostate cancers, one rectal cancer and bladder cancer, one histiocytoma in the 90-mg group.
[b] Millimeters on visual analogue scale.

Results

Pain Intensity

Patients randomized to the 60-mg group and the 90-mg group reduced their mean value of pain intensity by 7.2±3.6 ($p=0.083$) and 7.1±4.9 ($p=0.296$) after the first infusion and by 12.21±4.7 ($p=0.0164$) and 16.9±3.8 ($p=0.0003$) after the third infusion, respectively. After the third infusion, the percent reduction in the 60-mg group was 23.75%, in the 90-mg group 29.83%. The difference between the treatment groups was not significant (Wilcoxon signed rank test: $p=0.829$). At the time of the sixth infusion (after five infusions) there were still significant reductions of pain intensity in both treatment groups of 20.39±4.8 and 12.5±5.1, respectively. The difference between the treatment groups was not significant (Wilcoxon signed rank test: $p=0.254$).

To estimate the overall benefit during treatment, the Wilcoxon signed rank test was used for comparison of the mean reduction of each treatment versus baseline values. No significant difference was found between treatment with

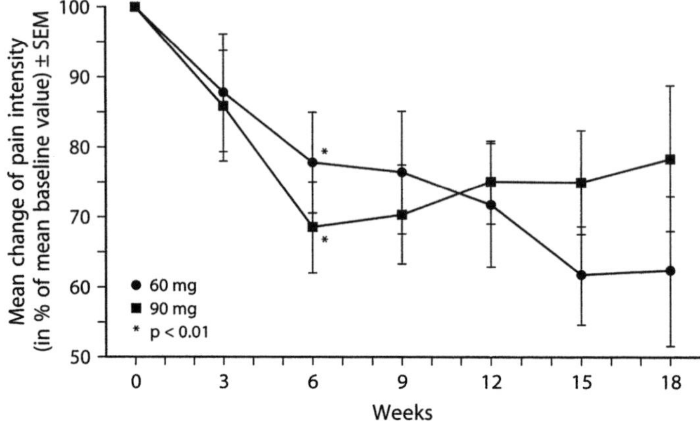

Fig. 17. Effects of pamidronate treatment on pain intensity in SG 110/93 protocol

60 mg and with 90 mg pamidronate every 3 weeks ($p=0.46$). See also Fig. 17. Asterix indicates earliest visit with significant difference of study parameter compared to baseline value.

Responders/Nonresponders

If a responder to treatment is defined as an individual with 10% or more reduction in pain intensity with pamidronate in comparison to her/his baseline value, then there is a clear increase in the proportion of responders with continuation of the treatment. There were 45% responders in the 60-mg group after the first infusion, 66% after the third infusion, and 78% after the fifth infusion. In the 90-g group the figures were 44%, 71%, and 63%, respectively. There was again no difference between the treatment arms at any of these time points using chi-square analysis. There were also no obvious differences between the two treatment groups with regard to subgroup analysis according to diagnosis.

Using the same criteria for response to pamidronate treatment, no differences were found between patients with progressive disease and those with stable disease, whereas all three patients who achieved partial remission responded after the first infusion and maintained the response throughout the study period.

If an overall mean reduction of 20 and more in the LASA scale of pain intensity is used as cut-off to define "pain response" as compared with the patient's baseline value, six of eight patients (75%) with multiple myeloma experienced clear-cut pain relief throughout the study period, whereas this was achieved in only 16 of 38 patients (42%) with solid tumors.

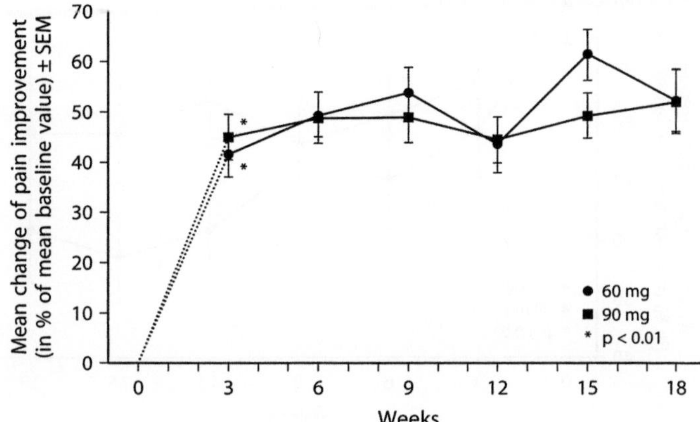

Fig. 18. Effects of pamidronate treatment on pain improvement in SG 110/93 protocol

Pain Improvement

After the first infusion pain improvement by 8.1 ($p=0.04$) in the lower-dose treatment group and 19.9 ($p=0.001$) in the higher-dose treatment group was noted. The respective figures after three and five infusions were 20.5 and 25.8 in the 60-mg group and 21.2 and 21.8 in the 90-mg group. There was a trend towards a better outcome in pain improvement with 90 mg pamidronate (median LASA 48) as compared with 60 mg (median LASA 34, $p=0.18$). The overall difference between the treatment arms favored the higher dose, but was again not significant ($p=0.173$). Mean changes in percent of pain improvement over time can be seen in Fig. 18. Asterix indicates earliest visit with significant difference of study parameter compared to baseline value.

Pain Frequency

Pain frequency at baseline was around 63 in both treatment groups and was reduced after one infusion by 13.8 in the 60-mg group and by 9.4 in the 90-mg group. The respective reductions after three infusions were 18.8 ($p=0.0014$) and 15.9 ($p=0.003$). A significant reduction of pain frequency was maintained with continuation of the treatment throughout the study period. The mean reduction in was 31.3 ($p=0.001$) the 60-mg arm and 15.8 ($p=0.0013$) in the 90-mg arm. The overall reduction throughout the study period was greater in the group of patients treated with 60 mg as compared with the patients treated with 90 mg ($p=0.0277$). Details can be seen in Fig. 19. Asterix indicates earliest visit with significant difference of study parameter compared to baseline value.

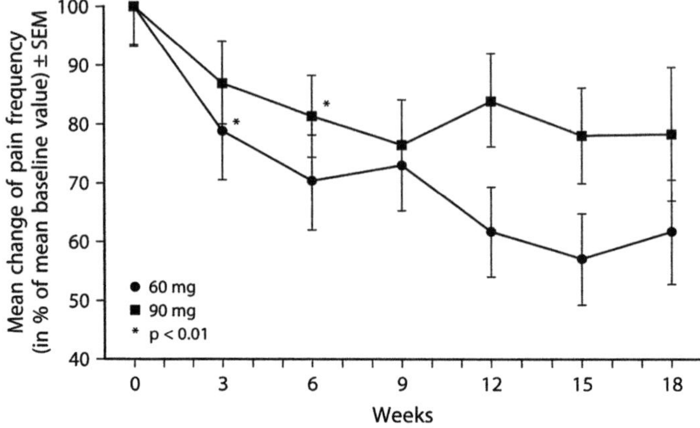

Fig. 19. Effects of pamidronate treatment on pain frequency in SG 110/93 protocol

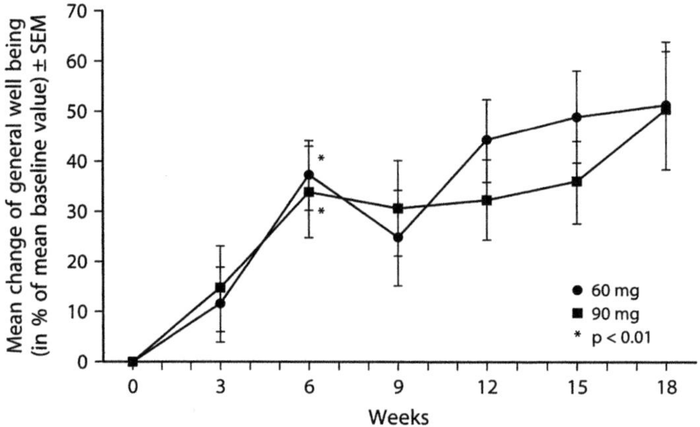

Fig. 20. Effects of pamidronate treatment on general well-being in SG 110/93 protocol

General Well-being

The mean baseline value for general well-being in the 60-mg group was 42.4 and in the 90-mg group 41.2. After the first infusion there was a small non-significant improvement in general well-being with both treatments. After three infusions the improvement in general well-being was 10.2 ($p=0.053$) in the 60-mg group and 11.3 ($p=0.086$) in the 90-mg group. After five infusions the respective figures were 17.1 ($p=0.014$) and 8.6 ($p=0.144$). The overall difference between the two treatment groups was not statistically significant ($p=0.116$). Changes in general well-being can be seen in Fig. 20. Asterix indicates earliest visit with significant difference of study parameter compared to baseline value.

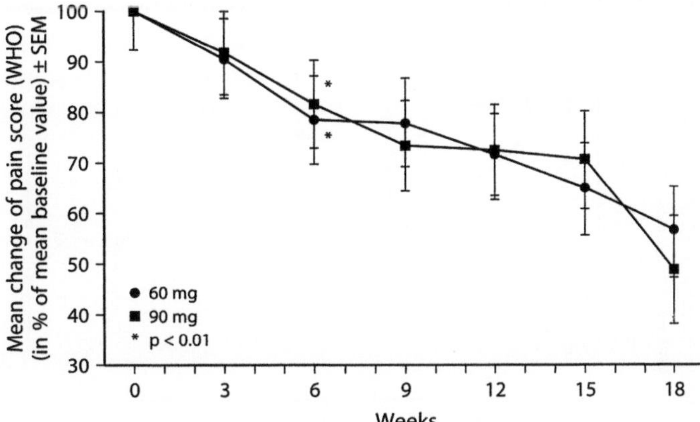

Fig. 21. Effects of pamidronate treatment on WHO pain score in SG 110/93 protocol

Pain Score

The mean pain score at baseline for patients randomized to the 60-mg group was 2.03±0.02, in those randomized to 90 mg pamidronate 2.17±0.2. There was a small reduction after the first treatment (–0.15 and –0.21). A greater reduction was noted after three infusions in both treatment arms: –0.45 ($p=0.017$) and –0.60±0.2 ($p=0.09$) respectively. The mean improvement in pain score after five infusions was 0.76±0.2 in the 60-mg group ($p=0.002$) and 0.46±0.3 ($p=0.080$) in the 90-mg group. The overall difference between the treatment arms throughout the study period was not significant ($p=0.67$). See also Fig. 21. Asterix indicates earliest visit with significant difference of study parameter compared to baseline value. As reported for the analgesic score, patients were categorized into groups, with improvement of one score, remaining at the same pain score level throughout the study period, or a worse pain score. The respective figures of the lower and the higher dose group were 8/23/4 and 8/22/4 after the first infusion, 14/10/5 and 15/10/5 after three infusions, and 15/8/2 and 11/9/6 after five infusions. Using the chi-square test for comparison of treatments and baseline proportions adjusted for baseline to the number of observations, there was a statistically significant improvement of mean pain score for both treatment groups at each time point measured throughout the study period. All p-values were ≤0.001.

Performance Status

The mean performance status at study entry was 1.51±0.2 for patients randomized to 60 mg and 1.69±0.2 for those randomized to 90 mg pamidronate. There was a small nonsignificant improvement in PS for patients treated with 60 mg, whereas PS in the 90-mg group virtually did not change throughout the study period. The difference between the 60-mg group and

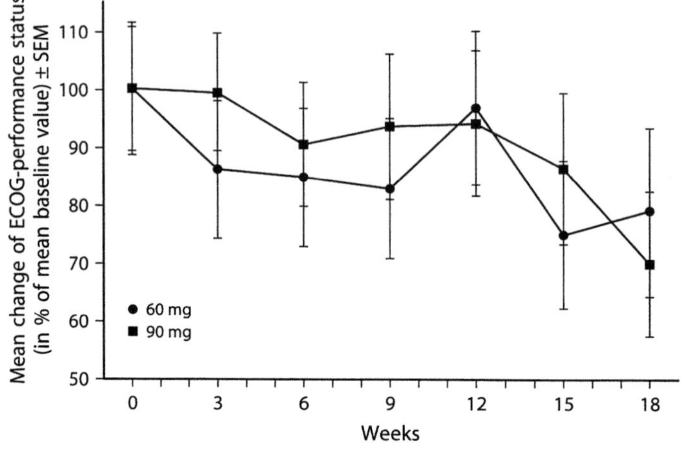

Fig. 22. Effects of pamidronate treatment on ECOG performance status in SG 110/93 protocol

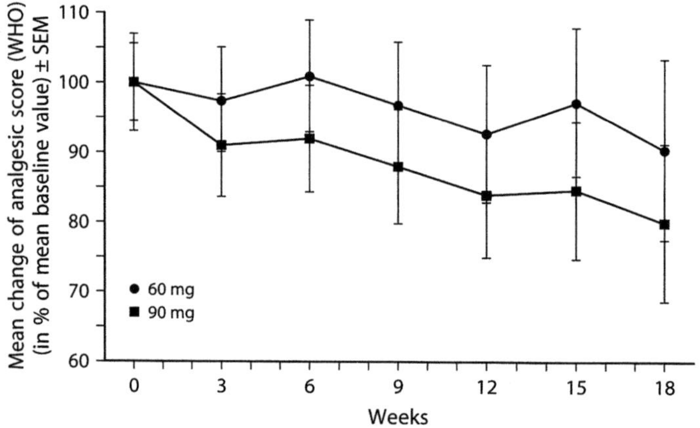

Fig. 23. Effects of pamidronate treatment on WHO analgesic score in SG 110/93 protocol

the 90-mg group reached statistical significance in favor of the 60-mg group ($p = 0.027$). However, as changes are also dependent on baseline values, the somewhat better baseline PS in the 60-mg group may have contributed to the overall result. See also Fig. 22.

When patients are categorized into groups according to improvement, no change, and worsening of PS, the figures for the 60-mg group and the 90-mg group were 6/26/1 and 4/24/6 ($p = 0.133$) after one infusion, 7/17/4 and 8/14/9 after three infusions, and 7/14/2 and 7/10/9 after five infusions, respectively. When the chi-square test for comparison of treatment and baseline proportions, adjusted for baseline to the number of observations, was performed, there were again statistically significant differences after one, three, and five infusions in both treatment arms ($p \leq 0.02$) but no significant differences between the treatment arms.

Analgesic Score

Mean analgesic score at baseline was 2.91±0.2 in the 60-mg group and 3.23±0.2 in the 90-mg group. Throughout the study period there was a small nonsignificant mean change in both groups towards consumption of less potent analgesics. The mean change in the 90-mg group was greater after one, three, and five infusions, which resulted in a significant difference in favor of the patients treated with 90 mg pamidronate ($p = 0.027$). Changes in analgesic score over time are shown in Fig. 23.

To gain further information, the patients were categorized into groups of those who improved (lowered) their level of analgesics, those who remained at the same level throughout the study period, and those who had to add a more potent group of analgesics for pain control to the already ongoing medication.

After the first infusion, the respective figures in the 60-mg group were 2/28/2 and in the 90-mg group 5/27/2, after three infusions 5/18/4 and 8/18/5, and after five infusions 4/14/6 and 7/16/3. There was no significant difference between the treatment groups at all these points in time. However, if comparison of treatment and baseline proportions, adjusted for baseline to the number of observations in the respective treatment groups, was made and the chi-square test for analysis of significance was performed, the figures showed a highly significant reduction of analgesics ($p \leq 0.02$) throughout the treatment period except for patients in the 60-mg group after the first infusion ($p = 0.118$).

Total Bone Mineral Density

Baseline values for total bone mineral density (mg/cm^2) at study entry were 1.112±0.2 in the 60-mg group and 1.074±0.3 in the 90-mg group. After three infusions there was a strong trend to higher bone mineral density in both arms with values of 1.144±0.2 ($p = 0.0494$) in the 60-mg group and 1.112±0.3 ($p = 0.0734$) in the 90-mg group. After six infusions there was a statistically significant increase only in the group of patients treated with 90 mg pamidronate. The respective figures were 1.121±0.3 ($p = 0.0837$) in the 60-mg group and 1.103±0.3 ($p = 0.0029$) in the 90-mg group; if one patient suffering from multiple myeloma, receiving successful chemotherapy, and achieving an extraordinary increase in bone mineral density from baseline value of 1.092 up to 1.330 (21.8%) at the termination of the treatment is excluded from the analysis, the increase of bone mineral density seen after three infusions disappears completely after six infusions for the 60-mg group as a whole. The respective figure for this group after six infusions drops to 1.112±0.2.

As far as percent change from baseline value is concerned, there was an increase in bone mineral density in the 60-mg group of 2.88% after three infusions and of 0.81% (all patients included in the analysis) at the end of the study period (Fig. 24). The respective figures in the 90-mg group are much

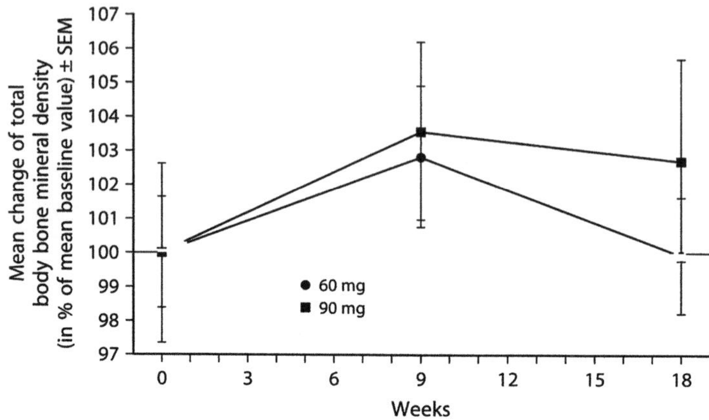

Fig. 24. Effects of pamidronate treatment on total body bone mineral density in SG 110/93 protocol

greater at 3.54% and 2.70%, which is a statistically significant increase versus baseline and significantly higher compared with patients who received 60 mg pamidronate ($p = 0.0286$).

When patients are categorized into groups with increased and decreased bone mineral density, the figures for patients treated with 60 mg were 12/5 after three infusions and 15/9 at the completion of pamidronate treatment. The respective figures in the 90-mg group are or were 10/5 and 14/2. Chi-square analysis for differences in the above-mentioned categories between the treatment groups were $p = 0.81$ after three infusions and $p = 0.083$ after six infusions.

Correlation of Results from Selected End Points

Pain Intensity and Bone Mineral Density

The correlation between "responders" and "nonresponders" in pain intensity was analyzed (for definition of response see section "Analysis of Pain Intensity"), as was that between categories of patients with increased and decreased bone mineral density during treatment.

After baseline values of bone mineral density were determined, 71 additional measurements were obtained during the study period, 40 in the 60-mg group and 31 in the 90-mg group.

In 49 cases an increased bone mineral density was measured, 25 in the 60-mg group and 24 in the 90-mg group. Based on these 49 measurements of increased bone mineral density, 33 patients were identified as responders (67%) and 16 were classified as nonresponders (33%). Among the 22 cases with decreased bone mineral density 17 patients were classified as responders (77%) and five (23%) as nonresponders.

We also performed a linear regression analysis, as well as Spearman's rank correlation of pain intensity versus bone mineral density, and found only a low regression coefficient with both treatments after three and after six infusions using both methods for analysis. r-Values using simple regression were below 0.455, the respective p-values $\geqslant 0.12$. Significance tests for Spearman's rank correlation showed p-values $\geqslant 0.24$.

Correlation of Bone Mineral Density and Diagnosis

Twelve of 17 patients with breast cancer had increased bone mineral density with 60 mg pamidronate, whereas eight of nine patients had increased bone mineral density with 90 mg pamidronate. Overall, there were 20 patients with breast cancer whose bone mineral density increased during treatment, whereas six patients had decreased bone mineral density. Eight of 13 multiple myeloma patients and eight of ten patients with tumors other than breast cancer or multiple myeloma showed increased bone mineral density.

Discussion

Our study population had very advanced malignant disease. Most patients also had progressive disease, either with ongoing treatment or without systemic antineoplastic treatment. Patients also had considerable pain, with a mean pain score of 2.4 despite the fact that the mean analgesic consumption reached a level of 3.4 on our modified WHO analgesic score. This means that our patient population usually used an opioid such as tramadol, codeine, or tilidine, in addition to full-dose nonsteroidal anti-inflammatory drugs such as 200 mg diclofenac per day or 1800–2400 mg ibuprofen per day. As a rule, in our institution analgesics are prescribed according to WHO guidelines (by the WHO ladder, by mouth, by the clock). Subjective pain assessment by LASA scales correlated well with the physicians' pain estimate using the WHO pain score. Both parameters showed clinically relevant residual pain at study entry. With regard to age and diagnoses, the patient population was similar to the one in our previously undertaken dose-escalation study. The results of this randomized study testing 60 mg versus 90 mg pamidronate given intravenously every 3 weeks confirmed our previous experience with pamidronate, which indicated a valuable palliative effect if the drug is used with adequate dose intensity. Both treatment arms showed a significant improvement in pain intensity, pain frequency, and general well-being, as rated by the patients. The changes in the LASA scales were slightly better for patients treated with pamidronate 90 mg. However, neither the randomized unblinded (SG 99/91) nor the randomized double-blind study (SG 100/93) was able to find a statistically significant difference between the treatment arms. There seems to be a trend in favor of 90 mg pamidronate in some parameters, such as bone mineral density, but this difference did not translate into a better palliative effect.

The overall results of our dose-escalation and randomized dose-seeking studies performed over a total of 8 years lead us to conclude that pamidronate given as repeated intravenous infusions to patients with advanced osteolytic bone disease and pain is an effective palliative treatment with regard to pain control and other quality-of-life parameters. A minimal single dose >30 mg and a dose intensity of at least 15 mg per week has to be administered to achieve a meaningful palliative effect. Tolererance is usually excellent. The palliative effect of pamidronate treatment might be greater in patients with multiple myeloma than in patients suffering from bone metastases of solid tumors. This view is supported by data obtained from indirect comparisons of placebo-controlled pamidronate studies, which will be discussed in the chapter "Recent Developments". In our study we found no consistent pattern of pain intensity and bone mineral density. It therefore remains necessary to investigate the clinically relevant patient-assessed parameters in future studies. Surrogate end points such as biochemical markers or bone mineral density are unreliable for estimating the impact of bisphosphonate treatment on the relevant quality-of-life parameters of patients with malignant osteolytic bone disease.

Similar conclusions have been drawn by A. Lipton et al. in the only other study that addressed the question of dose-effect relationship of pamidronate in a prospective randomized trial of patients with advanced breast and prostate cancer. Details have been described in the previous sections. No further data are available.

The dose-effect relationship of clodronate has been investigated with regard to inhibition of bone resorption. This study tested the effect of placebo, 400 mg, 1600 mg, or 3200 mg of oral clodronate administered daily for 4 weeks. The primary end point was the change of fasting urinary calcium excretion, expressed as the ratio of calcium/creatinine ratio in the fasting second-spot urine sample. Patients with fasting urinary calcium excretion <0.175 µmol/µmol creatinine or with a change of antineoplastic treatment within 1 month prior to the start of the trial or during the trial period were excluded from the trial. Eighty of 84 patients included in the trial completed the study. Sixty-nine patients had breast cancer. Median age was 57 years. Treatment adherence was monitored by weekly pill count and by high-performence liquid chromatography on serum samples taken at baseline and after 4 weeks of clodronate treatment. Compliance was >99% by pill count, and serum clodronate levels at week 4 were 0 ng/ml, 69 ng/ml, 450 ng/ml, and 1770 ng/ml in the placebo, 400-mg, 1600-mg, and 3200-mg groups, respectively. The results demonstrated a dose-dependent reduction of calcium excretion in the clodronate groups, which became apparent within 1 week of treatment at doses of 1600 mg and 3200 mg daily. After 4 weeks the mean calcium excretion was virtually unchanged in the 400-mg group but significantly decreased in the 1600-mg and 3200-mg groups. In contrast, calcium excretion in the placebo group increased to 37% of baseline values after

4 weeks. Urinary hydroxyproline excretion showed similar trends. Bone alkaline phosphatase activity, indicating bone repair, increased significantly in the 1600-mg and 3200-mg groups, but changes in the 400-mg and placebo groups were not statistically different from the baseline values. Pain was assessed weekly using LASA scales, and analgesic intake was also documented weekly. The majority of patients (73%) were on analgesic drugs at study entry. No correlation between pain and either number of bone metastases or degree of bone resorption estimated by fasting calcium excretion was found at study entry. After 4 weeks of treatment the analgesic requirement remained unchanged. LASA pain values were also without significant changes within or between the treatment groups throughout the study period. Tolerance was excellent, with the exception of flatulence, which was reported in all clodronate groups but not in the placebo group. The authors conclude that a dose of 1600 mg clodronate is appropriate for long-term treatment. With regard to inhibition of bone resorption, there seems to be a threshold at this dose level, above which the dose-effect curve flattens and more pronounced effects are seen in only certain parameters (O'Rourke et al. 1995).

These results are confirmed by several studies testing oral ibandronate in patients with breast cancer and bone metastases. These studies showed that bone resorption measured by fasting calcium excretion and other parameters could be successfully inhibited, but doses of 20 mg oral ibandronate daily were as effective as doses of 50 mg daily (Boehringer Mannheim: data on file).

The results of the above-mentioned oral clodronate dose-response study from the United Kingdom and the international multicenter study of ibandronate are in line with our results. They show an upper threshold for inhibition of bone resorption in patients with malignancies and osteolytic bone disease. The failure to detect a difference in LASA pain values or analgesic requirements is most probably explained by the short treatment duration of 4 weeks in both studies. Neither study was designed to search for differences in the palliative effect.

The degree of inhibition of bone resorption with a 4-week oral treatment of clodronate is too low to achieve a clinically measurable palliative effect. This view is supported by studies of Adami and co-workers, who found no effect of oral clodronate after 2 weeks, but a marked decrease of pain and analgesic intake after a 2-week treatment with intravenous clodronate (Adami and Mian 1989). The results with 4 weeks of oral ibandronate, a much more potent bisphosphonate, are different. The degree of inhibition of bone resorption is similar to that obtained with the usual 2-mg bolus injection. Dose escalation with intravenous ibandronate also showed an upper threshold for inhibition of bone resorption. Prospective randomized double-blind, placebo-controlled studies of intravenous doses up to 6 mg ibandronate every 4 weeks to investigate dose effects on quality of life and laboratory parameters in patients with breast cancer, prostate cancer, and multiple myeloma are ongoing or already closed for accrual. No results of these studies are available so far.

Our studies with repeated infusions of pamidronate showed no difference in inhibition of bone resorption as measured by fasting calcium excretion with single doses of 60 mg and 90 mg. As shown in other studies using intravenous pamidronate (by Lipton and co-workers) and other bisphosphonates, there is a dose-effect relationship, but doses higher than 60 mg given intravenously every 3 weeks are not more effective for the palliation of advanced malignancy and painful osteolytic bone destruction. Higher doses of 90 mg showed a trend to increased bone mineral density, but this effect did not translate into a clinical improvement of the patients' quality of life. The threshold is most probably explained by mechanisms which lead to pain and other symptoms without an association to malignant osteolysis. These mechanisms include microfractures, nerve compression, and bending of the periosteum due to extension of bone metastases and other factors. Potent analgesics can also impair the patients' quality of life. Furthermore, many of these patients also have extraosseous tumor manifestations, which can cause pain and are not improved by bisphosphonate treatment. It is interesting to note that in our study SG 110/93 better pain control was achieved in patients with myeloma than in patients with metastatic solid tumors.

References

Adami S, Mian M (1989) Clodronate therapy of metastatic bone disease in patients with prostatic carcinoma. In: Herfarth C, Senn HJ (eds) Recent results in cancer research, vol 116. Springer, Berlin Heidelberg New York, pp 67–72

O'Rourke N, McCloskey E, Houghton F, Huss H, Kanis JA (1995) Double-blind, placebo-controlled, dose-response trial of oral clodronate in patients with bone metastases. J Clin Oncol 13:929–934

Cost-Effectiveness Analysis of Pamidronate Treatment in Patients with Advanced Malignant Osteolytic Bone Disease: SG 110/93 Plus

Introduction

Considerations of cost-effectiveness play a major role when new treatments are introduced for diseases in which other treatment modalities have an established role. Usually, the new modalities lead to extra costs, as they are given rather as an additive than as a replacement of established therapies. We therefore also explored this field of bisphosphonate treatment in a prospective pharmacoeconomic study in conjunction with the Research Group on Management in the Health System University of St. Gallen, Switzerland.

The objective of this economic study was to analyze the consequences of two different dosages of Aredia on the cost-effectiveness relationship of the treatment. The study was added on to a clinical trial conducted as a randomized, double-blind phase-II study investigating the effectiveness of 60 mg vs. 90 mg of Aredia in patients with malignant tumors, osteolytic bone diseases, and pain (clinical trial SG 110/93).

In particular, the objectives of the economic study were (a) to assess the economic consequences of the Aredia treatment alongside a clinical trial in a prospective way, and thus (b) to provide a base for the evaluation of a cost-effectiveness relationship of the drug administered at two dosage levels for the treatment of patients with malignant osteolytic bone disease. Thus, the basic question to be answered was whether it "paid" to prescribe 90 mg of Aredia. Concomitantly, a more general goal was to show that economic evaluations may be conducted efficiently alongside clinical studies.

Patients and Methods

The analysis of direct costs of patient care during Aredia® treatment and during follow-up were based on data concerning the total charges – used as proxies for costs – for all outpatient care and all inpatient care. The approximation of costs by charges was justified because differences in costs (between the 60-mg and the 90-mg group) were focused on and since all patients were treated at one medical center (guaranteeing consistency of data). Three groups of effectiveness parameters were observed and analyzed. The first pertained to avoidance of institutionalization as expressed by hospitalization rates and number of inpatient days. The second related to avoidance of therapy of complications, i.e., radiation therapy – omitting the planned analysis of occurrence of orthopedic surgery because of zero values. The third evaluated measures of well-being of the patients as expressed by their own judgement of pain intensity. During the treatment phase, the patient samples comprised 28 cases in the 60-mg Aredia® group and 27 cases in the 90-mg group. The average age in both groups was approximately 62 years. Two thirds of the patients were breast cancer cases, about a fifth had multiple myelomas, and the rest included other tumors.

Results

The average costs (charges) per patient of the two patient samples did not differ. The total costs incurred during the Aredia® treatment phase plus the 6-month follow-up phase amounted to approximately 18,000 SFr for the group administered 60 mg Aredia® and 24,000 SFr for the 90-mg group (calculated on the basis of the median values in both groups; difference statistically not significant). The treatment phase was slightly more costly than the 6-month follow-up. The average patient incurred charges of approximately 2000 SFr per month during the 4-month treatment phase. During follow-up the monthly costs amounted to approximately 1700 SFr. The differences between the samples were, in both phases, statistically not significant.

The effectiveness measures analyzed during Aredia® treatment plus 1 year of follow-up showed no differences in hospitalization rates between the samples, approximately 45% of the patients being referred to hospital. The duration of hospitalization was equal in both samples, too. The patients were hospitalized for approximately 5 days per month. Analogous results were obtained for the avoidance of radiotherapy. Approximately half of the patients were prescribed radiotherapy in both groups. On average, those prescribed radiotherapy were treated on about 1.4 days per month. There were no statistically significant differences between the two patient groups.

The consequences of Aredia® were clear and significant in the analysis of pain intensity, which improved for both patient groups. After the first Aredia® administration both groups showed an improvement of approximately 15% (patient judgement on the LASA scale). After the third administration, the patients of the 60-mg group reported a larger improvement of about 20%, the 90-mg group approximately 30%. After the sixth and last administration, the 60-mg group was close to a 40% improvement, while the 90-mg group receded to a smaller improvement of approximately 20%. The lessening of pain was, within each group, statistically significant with respect to baseline. The differences between the groups were not significant, except for the last report.

Conclusion

The cost data of the patient samples were identical, i.e., independent of the dosage of Aredia® – at least for the average of the patients investigated. Among the effectiveness parameters, there was no difference between the two patient groups either (with the exception of pain intensity towards the end of the treatment period). It may be concluded that in this study the difference in dosages of Aredia® did not have any influence, either on costs or on the main effectiveness parameters.

Therefore, it was not attempted to define cost-to-effectiveness relations. It should be noted, however, that the particular patient samples studied may not have allowed for the detection of a possible smaller difference of the dosages. Thus, it is possible that the large variances in the observation and the heterogeneous patient population (different tumor types, different disease states, etc.) could obscure possible outcomes of interest – although the design and implementation of the study were nearly optimal. However, this study did not find a clinically relevant difference in the outcome for the two doses, and therefore the costs for the pamidronate treatment will have to be compared with the total costs that will be incurred for the disease management and the improvement of the quality of life of these patients. The cost for pamidronate was only about 10% of the total treatment costs that arose during the study treatment and observation period of 10 months – irrespective of whether pamidronate had been given in a dose of 60 or 90 mg every 3 weeks.

Recent Developments and Future Directions

Ibandronate

Ibandronate, a very potent third-generation compound, has been developed and clinically tested during the 1990s. Results of the two randomized, double-blind, three-arm studies (BM 21 0955 i.v. in tumor-induced hypercalcemia: SG 97/91 and SG 107/92) have been published recently and are summarized in the subsection "Bisphosphonates" of the section "Hypercalcemia of Malignancy". An oral formulation has been investigated in patients with breast cancer and bone metastases (SG 98/91). A dose-dependent inhibition of bone resorption was demonstrated, but occasional gastrointestinal side effects led to the development of a new oral formulation of ibandronate. Ibandronate was also tested as an intravenous bolus injection in tumor-induced osteolysis (SG 122/93). Again, a dose-dependent inhibition of bone resorption as measured by biochemical markers of bone turnover was found. Tolerance was excellent. Finally, a prospective, randomized, double-blind, placebo-controlled, three-arm, phase-III study of ibandronate has been conducted in patients with breast cancer and bone metastases (SG 143/94). No results are available to the public so far.

Pamidronate

Two pivotal studies of pamidronate were published in 1996, and results were submitted to the state authorities for registration of the drug for use in patients with advanced myeloma (Berenson et al. 1996) and in patients with advanced breast cancer and lytic bone metastases (Hortobagyi et al. 1996). Both phase-III studies randomized a large number of patients to either placebo or pamidronate 90 mg given every 4 weeks. The treatment was given as a 4-h intravenous infusion for nine cycles in the myeloma trial and as a 2-h intravenous infusion for 12 cycles in the breast cancer trial. In the first study, patients with stage III multiple myeloma and creatinine <442 mol/l and adequate organ function were eligible. Patients were stratified at study entry for first-line chemotherapy (stratum 1) versus second-line chemotherapy (stratum 2); 392 patients were included in the study. Results showed that the proportion of patients with skeletal events was significantly lower in the pamidronate group (24%) compared with the placebo group (41%, $p<0.001$). This reduction was evident in both stratum 1 ($p=0.04$) and stratum 2 ($p=0.004$). Patients receiving pamidronate also had a significant decrease in bone pain and no deterioration in overall performance status and quality-of-life parameters. In this study clinically relevant skeletal events were investigated; occurrence of hypercalcemia was not regarded as a clinically meaningful event, in contrast to most other placebo-controlled bisphosphonate trials in malignant osteolytic bone disease that have been performed up to now. Despite this stringent implementation of study end points, the benefit in the pamidronate group was seen throughout the analyzed study period, from the time of randomization through March 1, 1994. The same was true for the reduction of radiation treatment to bone. Pathological fractures were increasingly reduced with continuation of the treatment. Overall, there were 50 vertebral and 20 nonvertebral fractures in the pamidronate group, as compared with 91 and 44, respectively, in the placebo group. The analysis of skeletal events according to stratum by the end of nine treatment cycles showed that pamidronate reduced the above-mentioned skeletal complications in both strata; pathological fractures were practically avoided in stratum 1 and to a lesser extent in stratum 2. The need for radiation treatment to bone was reduced by almost 50% in stratum 2, whereas patients with less advanced disease (in stratum 1) had no reduction in the frequency of radiation treatment to bone. The serum and urinary markers of both bone resorption and bone formation were reduced in the pamidronate group throughout the treatment period, but they did not change in the placebo group. The median decrease form baseline at the final measurement in the pamidronate group was 32% for the urinary calcium creatinine ratio and 26% for the urinary hydroxyproline creatinine ratio. In the pamidronate group alkaline-phosphatase decreased by 56% and serum osteocalcin by 50% at the final measurement. With a median follow-up of 17 months, the estimated median survival was 28 months in the pamidronate group and 23 months in the placebo group ($p=0.082$). Longer follow-up will show whether there is a real survival advantage for patients treated with pamidronate in additional to chemotherapy. A possible difference might be attributed to the reduction in complications of multiple myeloma by pamidronate treatment as demonstrated in this study. However, it is important to note that interleukin-6, an essential growth factor for myeloma cells, is produced by bone cells themselves, exerting their effect via a paracrine pathway (Bataille et al. 1992). Thus there is pathophysiological evidence of a vicious cycle involving myeloma cells and their stromal environment, with the former stimulating the latter to resorb bone. Osteoclastic bone resorption leads to the release of factors which also support tumor growth. Inhibition of bone resorption could therefore also inhibit the growth of myeloma cells. Bisphosphonates can inhibit the production of interleukin-6 by osteoblasts (Passeri et al. 1994). Moreover, the inhibitory effect of bisphosphonates on Il-6 production is also suggested by their inhibitory action on monocyte proliferation (Baier 1995). Since monocyte stimulation is also mediated by Il-6, bisphosphonate-induced inhibition of monocyte growth (and their further development to mature osteoclasts) could also be explained, at least in part, by the inhibition of Il-6. Furthermore, pamidronate infusions also lowered the serum Il-6 levels in cancer patients with bone metastases (Lissoni et al. 1997). The aforementioned cascade also explains another pathway of inhibition of bone breakdown by osteoclasts alongside the more commonly known direct inhibition of the mature osteoclast, at least in myeloma patients.

The second pivotal study included 382 women with advanced breast cancer and lytic metastatic bone lesions, one of which was at least 1 cm in diameter. Patients had to have adequate organ functions. Patients with pathological fractures, needing radiation or bone surgery, or having spinal compression and hypercalcemia at the time of study entry were not eligible. The presence of a lytic lesion that could be evaluated was confirmed by a central radiologist. During the trial, the chemotherapy regimen could be changed or discontinued at the discretion of the attending physician. Data on efficacy and safety were analyzed for the 12 cycles of the treatment period. Survival was followed until the patient's death, the last date of contact in case of loss to follow-up, or February 1, 1995, whichever occurred first. The clinical features at study entry were similar in the two groups regarding the number of prior chemotherapy regimens or hormone treatments, the use of analgesic drugs, and the quality-of-life scores. The frequency of prior treatment with chemotherapy regimens containing tamoxifen, megestrol acetate, aminoglutethimide, and doxorubicin were similar in both groups.

Forty-eight percent of the patients completed all 12 cycles of pamidronate or placebo. The mean duration of participation was 9.6 months in the pamidronate group and 8.9 months in the placebo group. The results showed that the median time to occurrence of the first skeletal complication in the pamidronate group was almost doubled as compared with the placebo group (13.1 vs. 7.0 months, $p=0.005$). Skeletal events (hypercalcemia again not included among the skeletal complications) occurred in 43% versus 56%, respectively ($p=0.008$). The increase in bone pain was significantly less ($p=0.046$), as was the deterioration of performance status ($p=0.027$) in patients treated with pamidronate. Nonvertebral pathological fractures, the need for radiation to bone, and surgery on bone, as well as the overall skeletal complications excluding hypercalcemia were significantly reduced after completion of the sixth cycle of pamidronate treatment. Pathological vertebral fractures and episodes of hypercalcemia were already significantly reduced after three infusions of pamidronate. Eighty-five percent of the patients also underwent radiological assessment at baseline and subsequently. Of these patients who could be evaluated radiologically, a significantly higher proportion showed complete or partial responses of lytic lesions in the pamidronate group than in the placebo group (33% versus 18%, $p=0.001$). Urinary calcium creatinine ratios decreased by 28% in the pamidronate group but increased by 25% in the placebo group. The respective values for urinary hydroxyproline-creatinine ratio are –33% and –6%, whereas serum bone alkaline phosphates decreased by 41% and 1% in the pamidronate treated group and the placebo group, respectively. The difference between the treatment groups for each variable was significant ($p<0.001$). The median estimated overall survival was 14.8 months in the pamidronate group and 14.2 months in the placebo group.

In conclusion, both studies showed that monthly infusions of 90 mg pamidronate constitute an effective additive treatment to chemotherapy for the reduction of skeletal complications and the relief of symptoms associated with lytic bone lesions due to multiple myeloma or breast cancer. Pamidronate was safe and well tolerated in both studies. Furthermore, a trend to better survival was observed in myeloma patients treated with pamidronate. The encouraging results show that potent bisphosphonates are important tools in the management of malignant osteolytic bone disease. The results of the breast cancer study also raise the question of whether bisphosphonates can delay or even prevent the occurrence of bone metastases in patients with breast cancer at high risk for developing bone metastases. Preclinical data showed that bisphosphonates can reduce the metastatic burden in the bone (Sasaki et al. 1995). These changes could be due to the inhibition of bone resorption. It is known that the release of growth factors stored in the bone matrix during bone degradation createsa favorable microenvironment for breast cancer cells to build a metastatic deposit. Furthermore, bisphosphonates were shown to inhibit the adhesion of breast cancer cells to the bone matrix in vitro (van der Pluijm et al. 1996).

Pioneering studies supporting this hypothesis were performed in the late 1980s by German experimental pathologists who pretreated rats with clodronate 30 mg/kg for 5 days, 4 weeks prior to intraosseous injection of Walker carcinosarcoma 256B cells. Ten days after the intraosseous injection, massive osteolytic destruction of the skeleton was seen in the control animals, whereas clodronate-pretreated animals had only a few small osteolytic lesions (Krempien et al. 1988; Krempien and Mangegold 1993).

Adjuvant Bisphosphonate Therapy

Several studies have shown that long-term supportive bisphosphonate treatment significantly reduces skeletal morbidity in patients with breast cancer and established metastatic bone disease and improves some selective aspects of quality of life. The question therefore arises whether bisphosphonate treatment initiated earlier during the course of disease, when the skeleton is free of bone metastases, can prevent or delay the development of bone involvement in patients at high risk for developing bone metastases.

Several attempts have been made to investigate this question and one study has recently been published. In an open prospective randomized study involving 124 patients with either extraskeletal metastases ($n=91$) or locally advanced disease ($n=33$) but no bone metastases at study entry, 56 patients received pamidronate given as enteric coated tablets of 150 mg to be taken with water twice daily 30 min before meals. Concomitant antineoplastic therapy was allowed. The median follow-up of the patients was 19 months with pamidronate and 24 months with control. This difference was due mainly to the refusal of 15 patients to continue pamidronate treatment because of gastrointestinal side effects. Fourteen of 65 patients (22%) and 12 of 59 patients (20%) developed a first skeletal event during the follow-up period in the pamidronate group and the control group, respectively. A comparison of the actuarial risk of a first skeletal event including hypercalcemia showed no significant difference ($p=0.57$). The cumulative incidence of first radiological skeletal events showed a trend which favored the control group ($p=0.15$). The reduction in quality of life as assessed by questionnaires was similar in both groups with regard to impairment of mobility, bone pain, gastrointestinal complaints, and fatigue.

This small study using oral pamidronate failed to show a beneficial effect of the adjuvant bisphosphonate treatment. However, the oral form of pamidronate is known to be associated with gastrointestinal toxicity, and the small study size does not allow firm conclusions on the (lack of) delay or prevention of metastatic bone involvement in breast cancer patients treated with adjuvant bisphosphonates (van Holten-Verzantvoort et al. 1996).

A second study using intravenous bisphosphonate, performed in the United Kingdom, has shown encouraging preliminary results, but no data based on a final analysis are available.

A Danish breast cancer study using oral pamidronate even earlier in the course of the disease – as adjuvant treatment to antineoplastic systemic treatment if indicated – has been performed with a large number of patients. However, due to the low number of bone events as first event, the study has not yet provided any conclusive results.

Kanis and co-workers randomized 133 women with recurrent breast cancer, but no evidence of skeletal metastases, to receive 1600 mg clodronate daily p.o. or an identical placebo for 3 years under double-blind conditions at two clinical oncology centers in the UK and Canada. The main measures of outcome included the occurrence of skeletal metastases, as judged from sequential bone scans and radiographs, and the morbidity associated with them, comprising the incidence of hypercalcemia, vertebral and nonvertebral fractures, and bone pain as assessed by the requirements for skeletal radiotherapy.

The number of patients who developed skeletal metastases was lower among clodronate-treated patients than among those who received the placebo (15 vs. 19) but was not significantly different. The number of skeletal metastases was significantly lower with clodronate than with placebo (32 vs. 63; $p<0.005$). The complications of skeletal disease were fewer by 26% in clodronate-treated patients compared with controls ($p<0.01$).

Compared with placebo, significant effects in favor of clodronate were observed for vertebral deformities (29%) and hypercalcemia (39%). There was no effect of clodronate on survival. It was concluded that clodronate given orally can significantly decrease the frequency of clinically overt skeletal metastases and can also decrease the morbidity associated therewith (Kanis et al. 1996).

Recently, I.J. Diel and co-workers presented preliminary data on 142 primary breast cancer patients with positive tumor cell detection in the bone marrow at the time of primary surgery. These patients received adjuvant treatment with the bisphosphate clodronate within a prospective randomized trial. At a median follow-up of 36 months, 21 patients in the clodronate group and 36 patients in the control group developed distant metastases ($p=0.007$). Bone metastases were more frequent in the control group than in the clodronate group, affecting 19 patients versus ten patients ($p=0.025$).These results are promising but need to be confirmed in larger multicenter studies (Diel et al. 1997).

Future Directions

Attempts have been made by several international breast cancer research groups to investigate the adjuvant use of more potent and less toxic bisphosphonates in patients with breast cancer at high risk of developing bone metastases. Further efforts will be necessary to identify those patients who will benefit most from bisphosphonate treatment both in the early, adjuvant, and in the late, palliative setting. Clinically relevant end points in an appropriate patient population have to be selected, and continuing progress with the existing methodology has to be made in order to enable treating physicians and health-care professionals to simplify the interpretation of the results of these trials. Patient and family well-being, patients' attitudes towards treatment, and continued confrontation with the disease by physician or hospital contacts, as well as direct and indirect costs, are new end points which have to be developed in these clinical trials. Resource allocation decisions will play a major role in health care in the future (Mc Vie et al. 1997).

New developments have facilitated the administration of these very potent third-generation compounds. They can be given as an intravenous bolus injection or as a short infusion. Excellent candidates for these investigations are ibandronate and zoledronate. The future will show whether such an organ-targeted adjuvant treatment can delay or prevent osteolytic bone metastases and thus improve the outcome of patients with cancer.

References

Baier JE (1995) Bisphosphonates – cellular mode of action. Influence on mediators within the immune system. Tumordiagn Ther 16:4–11

Bataille R, Capparad D, Klein B (1992) Mechanisms of bone lesion in multiple myeloma. Hematol Oncol Clin North Am 6:285–295

Berenson JR, Lichtenstein A, Porter L, et al (1996) Efficacy in reducing skeletal events in patients with advanced muliple myeloma. N Engl J Med 334:488–493

Diel IJ, Solomayer EF, Goerner R, Gollan C, Wallwiener D, Bastea G (1997) Adjuvant treatment of breast cancer patients with the bisphosphonate clodronate reduces incidence and number of bone and non-bone metastases. Am Soc Clin Oncol 16:abstract 461

Hortobagyi GN, Theriaut RL, Porter L, et al for the Protocol 19 Aredia® Breast Cancer Study Group (1996) Efficacy of pamidronate in reducing skeletal complications in patients with breast cancer and lytic bone metastases. N Engl J Med 335:1785–1791

Kanis JA, Powles T, Paterson AHG, MacCloskey EV, Ashley S (1996) Clodronate decreases the frequency of skeletal metastases in women with breast cancer. Bone 19:663–667

Krempien B, Mangegold C (1993) Prophylactic treatment of skeletal metastases, tumour-induced osteolysis, and hypercalcemia in rats with the bisphosphonate CL_2 MBP. Cancer 72:91–98

Krempien B, Wingen F, Eichmann T, Müller M, Schmähl D (1988) Protective effects of prophylactic treatment with the bisphosphonate 3-amino-1-hydroxypropane-1,1-bisphosphonic acid on the development of tumour osteopathy in the rat: experimental studies with the Walker carcinosarcoma 256. Oncology 45:41–46

Lissoni P, Cazzaniga M, Barni S, et al (1997) Acute effects of bisphosphonate agent disodium pamidronate administration on serum levels of interleukin-6 in advanced solid tumour patients with bone metastases and their possible implications in the immunotherapy of cancer with interleukin-2. Eur J Cancer 33:304–306

Mc Vie JG, Cvitkovic E, ten Bokkel Huinink W, Redmond K, MacRae K (1997) Response rate, survival or other endpoints? – a scientific debate. Eur J Cancer 33 [Suppl 2]:1–17

Passeri G, Ulietti V, Girasole G, et al (1994) Bisphosphonates inhibit IL-6 production by human osteoblastic cells MG-63. J Bone Miner Res 9:230 abstract

Sasaki A, Boyce BF, Story B, et al (1995) Bisphosphonate risedronate reduces metastatic human breast cancer burden in bone in nude mice. Cancer Res 55:3551–3557

van Holten-Verzantvoort ATM, Hermans J, Bex LVAM, et al (1996) Can supportive pamidronate treatment prevent or delay the first manifestation of bone metastases in breast cancer patients? Eur J Cancer 32A:450–454

van der Pluijm G, Vloedgraven H, Van Beck E, Van der Wee-Pals L, Lowik C, Papapoulos S (1996) Bisphosphonates inhibit the adhesion of breast cancer cells to bone matrices in vitro. J Clin Invest 98:698–705

Recent Results in Cancer Research
Volumes published since Vol. 146

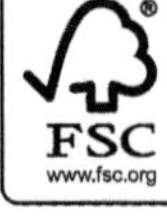